I0841236

Early praise for the book

"The authors have presented a unique method of employing simple graphics, rather than pie charts or line graphs, or a slew of statistical data, to present an in-depth analysis of medical treatment. In simple language, they have demonstrated how their Benefit-Risk Characterization Theatre (BRCT), which is a 1,000-seater theatre, the benefits and risks of any medical intervention can be clearly displayed in a simple manner. Policy makers as well the general population can benefit from this simple, easy-to-understand tool. This will be especially useful in the current times when the entire world is struggling with the COVID-19 pandemic and no one really knows for sure how to tackle the situation."

—Anmet Systems Editorial Staff

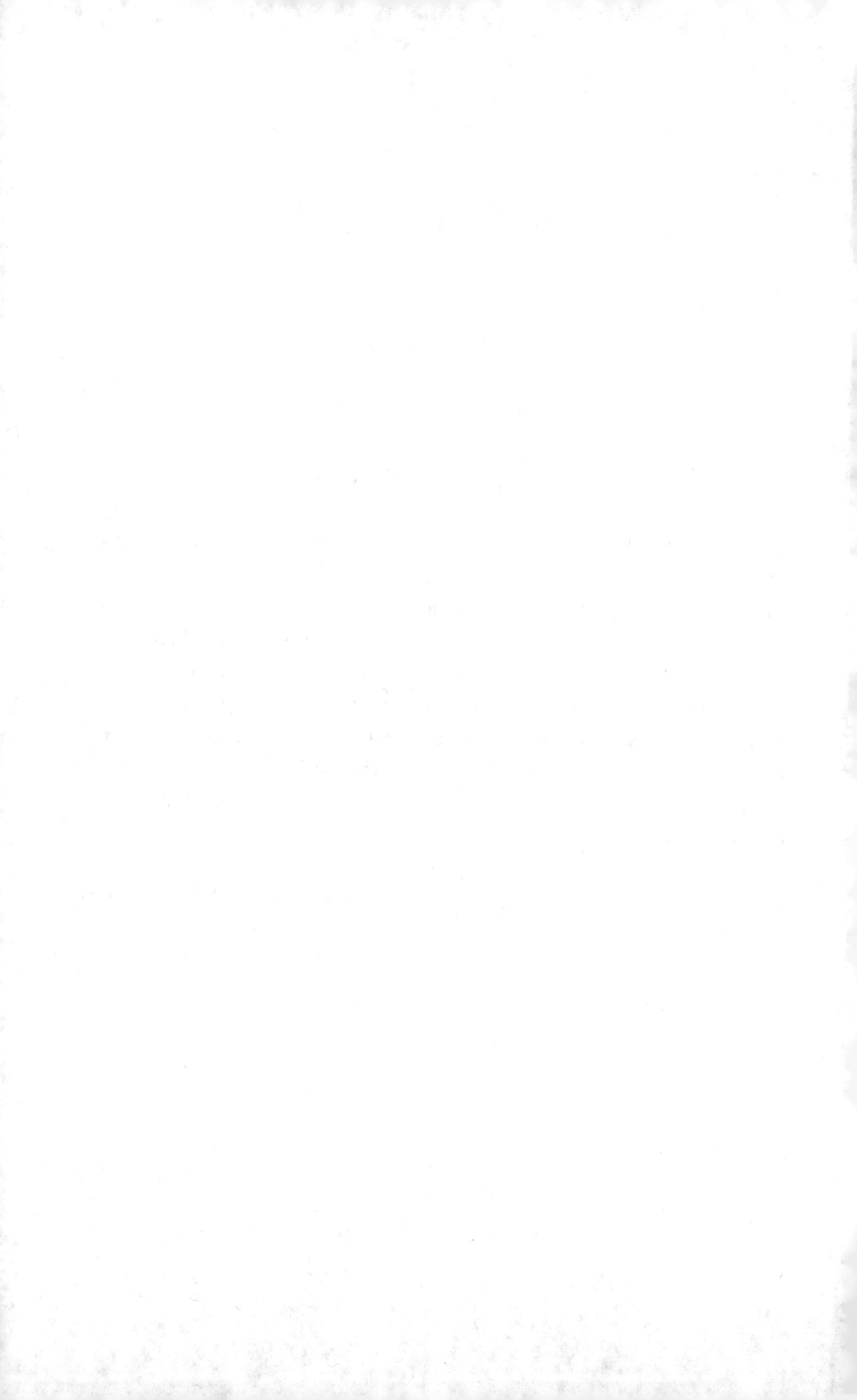

Understanding COVID-19 Risks: An Image Is Worth More Than 1,000 Words

Understanding COVID-19 Risks: An Image Is Worth More Than 1,000 Words

NOW IT'S UP TO YOU!

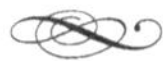

Andy Lazris, MD and Erik Rifkin, PhD

Copyright © 2021 Andy Lazris, MD and Erik Rifkin, PhD

All rights reserved.

ISBN-13:

Table of Contents

Preface

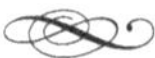

THE PRIMARY OBJECTIVE OF THIS book is to demonstrate how a simple graphic can be used to dramatically improve accurate communication of health risks from exposure to COVID-19, as well as to assess the measures we are undertaking to contain and treat the outbreak. To date, there have been far-reaching ramifications based on ineffective risk communication when attempting to clarify these health endpoints.

Another goal is to emphasize the importance and significance of using a standard visual approach to communicate information about a variety of health endpoints. Our previous book, *Interpreting Health Benefits and Risks*, published by Springer, used the same visual graphic across a spectrum of health endpoints. Research has demonstrated that information obtained visually is retained better than that obtained through text, equations, or complicated charts. It is also more accurate. Most of us have had this experience!

We are both experts in this field. Erik has a PhD and has worked extensively in environmental science, creating the Benefit-Risk Characterization Theater (BRCT) through which we have presented our data. Andy has an MD and is a primary care physician who has written numerous books on health care and who has been on the frontline of the COVID-19 outbreak, caring for hundreds of COVID-19 infected patients mostly in long-term care. Both of us have given countless talks, written articles, op-eds, and other academic books on the subject, and produced videos—all related to presenting health data in a BRCT context.

There are other reasons as to why we chose to write this book for the general public at this time:

- We are authors of a book to be published by Springer Nature In August 2021 (***Utilizing Effective Risk Communication in COVID-19 - Highlighting the BRCT***). It is also far more detailed and geared toward medical schools, scientists, and government agencies.
- There have been relevant events that happened after the text of the first book was completed (e.g., benefits and risks associated with vaccines for COVID-19).
- For many months, experts on viruses have been acknowledging, on TV and other media, that there is a critical need for improving accurate communication of COVID-19 risks. However, specific, meaningful suggestions have rarely followed. That is what this book is all about. We are responding to that call!
- The cost of this book should encourage the public, concerned about and interested in COVID-19, to learn more about the benefits of using our innovative concept to explain and solve problems.

Another goal is to demonstrate that health communication can be direct and straightforward if done correctly. The ramifications of poor health communication are apparent every day, but they were devastating during the past year of the COVID-19 pandemic. Because of poor communication, there was a cloud of fear, confusion, and uncertainty among the public and those trying to treat the disease.

This led to the implementation of measures that were not always effective and were sometimes harmful; as a result, misinformation was frequently portrayed as science. We hope to show in this short book that communication could have been far more accurate and easily understood by employing our simple graphic. And this approach can be used in future, similar situations.

In our previous work, much of which can be found on our website www.doc-patient-talk.com, we showed how virtually all health data can be incorporated into a theatrical representation of risk and benefit. Below is a BRCT, which is simply a 1,000-seat theater used to represent a group of people. The use of this BRCT will be demonstrated in the following chapters.

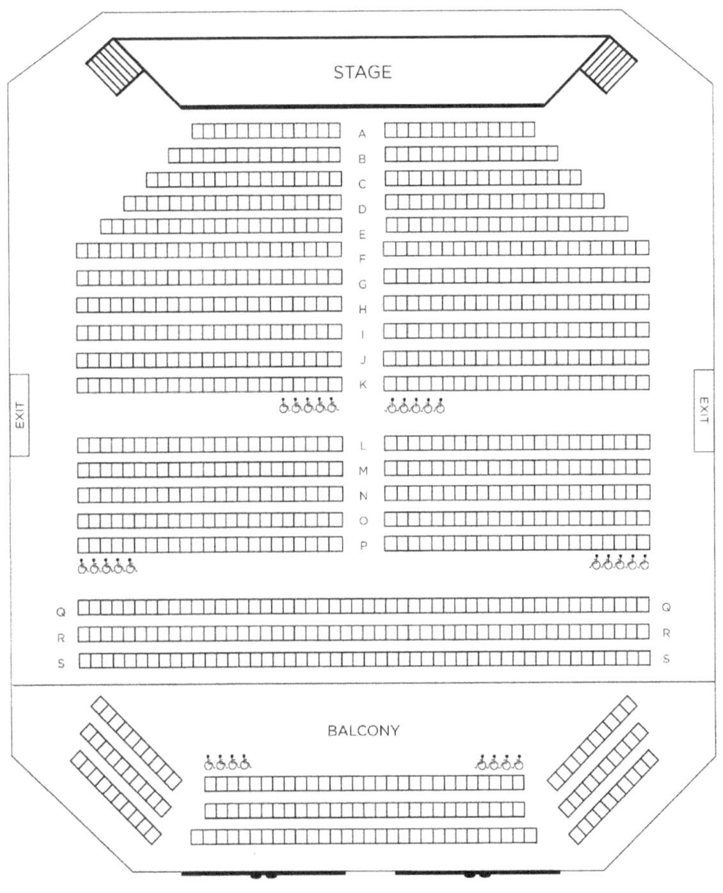

All health care data can be put into this theater to demonstrate the risks and benefits of treatments, as well as the risk of disease. The standard approach of flashing traditional pie charts or line graphs, which demand considerable statistical sophistication to fully understand, is not going to resonate with most folks—or physicians for that matter.

Most patients are not doctors or scientists. Equations, calculations, percentages, or technical text would add to their confusion. Since an image is worth thousands of words, what is needed is a simple, straightforward graphic that presents, on one page, a clear and objective picture of health benefits and risks associated with COVID-19 and other medical conditions.

Most of us are *familiar* with the crowd in a typical theater as a graphic illustration of a population grouping. It occurred to us that a theater seating chart could be used to objectively characterize and communicate health benefits and risks. We call this decision aid a *Benefit-Risk Characterization Theater (BRCT)©*. We have successfully used it to assist patients in determining their level of acceptable risk; if the benefits of intervention outweigh the risks, who should make the final decision regarding medical intervention; and whether the decision is evidence-based.

On our website, <u>several videos</u> use the BRCT to help clarify health decisions. For example, we <u>made a video</u> about a speculative wonder drug that is introduced to the market and touted as reducing one's chance of dying of a certain disease by 50 percent. But, what does that mean? Fifty percent of what? What are the risks of the drug? Usually, statistics can be confusing about the risks and benefits of most medical interventions such as these, but as is evident from the video, a **BRCT** helps facilitate your decision-making process about whether the "wonder drug" is right for you.

In the end, health decisions need to be made by every individual in a way that is appropriate to his or her own circumstances. Only by having accurate and easily understood data, though, can someone make an appropriate decision. The BRCT allows data to be presented in that way. We have used BRCTs in many endpoints, such as the following links below:

- Whether to treat sinusitis with antibiotics
- Whether to get an MRI for lower back pain
- Whether to get a mammogram (from NPR and Kaiser Health News)
- Various health endpoints, such as stents and lung cancer screening, as seen in our book

During the COVID-19 pandemic, communication could have been simplified and made more accurate using the BRCT. This could have helped people to better assess their own risks of COVID-19 and the best ways to protect themselves and their loved ones. It could have helped public health officials and policymakers to better understand and assess the measures being used to treat and contain the disease. We have used BRCTs to do just that in this book. Through them, we hope to

- significantly improve accurate communication of health risks from exposure to COVID-19, and
- assess how best to contain and control COVID-19.

Why all the confusion?

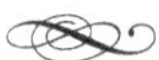

Poor communication during the first year of the COVID-19 pandemic has led to confusion, misinformation, inaccurate assessment of risk, and poor policy decisions. In essence, those who spoke about COVID-19 most publicly were often misleading in their dissemination of information or based their conclusions on an inaccurate interpretation of data or on poor data.

Experts vs. Facts. All through the pandemic, we heard from "experts" from federal or state agencies, academic centers, news outlets, or other prestigious institutions. The very fact that they, or the press, declared them to be experts seemed to excuse them from providing data to support what they were contending to be true.

Experts from different states, different countries, and on the media often declared contradictory "facts" to be true whether it was the benefit of wearing a mask, the need to close schools, the risks and benefits of vaccination, or even the need to keep society shut down for a year.

Any information given out about COVID-19 should have been backed by facts. Those facts should have informed which people were most at risk, whether certain interventions worked or perhaps caused harm, and **what we didn't know**. Yes, it is very important to acknowledge what we do not know. But far too often, no facts were used in the dissemination of information, and that led to confusion and misinformation, which led to policies that were based on speculation.

We have always stated that all medical data can be put into a BRCT, and if it can't be put into a BRCT, then we have insufficient or inaccurate data. In this book, we have looked at the facts regarding disease risk, as well as the risks and benefits of our "treatment" of the disease. In some chapters, we have theaters with seats to demonstrate what we know, and in other chapters, we have theaters with a **?** to show what we don't know. In any health-related communication, it is important to emphasize both what is known and what is unknown about a disease or the treatment of that disease. However, during the pandemic, such data was not used by the experts to buttress their claims. We hope to show how it could have been done and can be done in the future, for COVID-19 and any other health care decision-making.

Disease vs. Treatment: Very often during the pandemic, we heard that the spread of COVID-19 led to the closure of schools and our society and caused depression among people. When we assess the risks and benefits of both the disease and its treatment, it is crucial to separate the two. For instance, if we treat you for a disease, and the treatment gives you side effects, we don't ascribe those side effects to the disease. We say that those side effects are from the treatment. Only by knowing the risks of the disease and the risks and benefits of the treatment can we determine what the best treatment is.

Unfortunately, communication in COVID-19 did not adhere to these rules. Many experts and news outlets simply lumped all the horrific things that happened this year under the category *caused by COVID-19*. When we do this, we are unable to ascertain if our treatments (masks, school closures, quarantines, etc.) are helping or harming people and society.

School closings are not caused by COVID-19; they are caused by policies to try to contain COVID-19. Thus, any adverse effects from school closings need to be put in the category of "side effects of our treatment." We have attempted to do just this in our book, because with a BRCT it is easy to show what the disease causes and what the treatment does, and only then can we construct policies that mitigate a disease without harming people with our treatments.

Who is speaking for the science: At the end of this book, we have listed many of the agencies that have spoken authoritatively about COVID-19. It's a long list! Most of us have heard from the media, government spokesmen, the Centers for Disease Control (CDC), or the National Institute of Health (NIH) on a regular basis.

Did these groups always disseminate factual and/or similar information and present those facts in an accurate and understandable manner? Very often, the answer was no. Many agencies made statements about risk and declarations about how to contain the disease, without providing any data. As we will show in this book, often there was no data to support their claims, and when the data did exist, it was presented in a way that was not clear or accurate. As such, much of the public and those who make our policies were fed information that they could not interpret accurately and got confused.

Through a BRCT approach, all of this could have been avoided. Again, there is much we do not know, but that too can be presented in a BRCT, and it is crucial that authoritative figures and agencies, as well as the press, acknowledge what we know and don't know. How else can we and the society make good judgments about how to best protect ourselves from COVID-19?

The news media has had twenty-four-hour coverage about COVID-19, very often in a sensationalized way. While they derived their information from experts, rarely did they delve into the science of what we know and what we don't know. That led to horrific repercussions. We hope with this book we can demonstrate how to communicate information about COVID-19, and all medical issues, in a scientific and easily understood way. As we said, a picture is worth a thousand words!

The extensive documentation that we used to create our theaters is in our Springer book and can be reviewed there. We have chosen to keep this book brief and mostly pictorial. You'll see that it's pretty amazing how much information can be conveyed with just a few words!

Now it is your turn to understand the risks of COVID-19 to you and both the risks and benefits of how to treat the pandemic. You'll see what is known and what is not known, and you can come to your own conclusions about whether we are handling the pandemic in the most scientific and effective way possible. Only by knowing what works and what doesn't can we derive better solutions. After obtaining the facts, **it's your decision!**

What is your risk? And, how accurately did experts convey the individual risk of COVID-19?

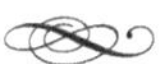

IN SUBSEQUENT CHAPTERS, WE WILL explore the risk of COVID-19 to the two extremes of age: 1) school-age kids and 2) elders in long-term care. Both groups sit on opposite poles of risk when it comes to serious consequences of COVID-19. However, in many ways, communication about COVID-19 failed to distinguish risk based on statistical data relating to the population within it (demographics).

In one sense, there was some fear that minimal and even asymptomatic infection in any person can lead to the dissemination of the virus to more high-risk groups. We saw, for instance, that when case rates increased in a community at large, then the case rate among people in long-term care concurrently went up, likely because people who work in long-term care also live in the community.

However, unless communication clearly defines the risk of disease between particular groups, people won't be aware of their individual risk from the disease and cannot react accordingly. And, policymakers cannot frame effective solutions to ease the impact of COVID-19 in a way that helps the vulnerable and does not harm those less at risk.

Throughout this crisis, various experts, government agencies, and media outlets have portrayed risk as being universal. News focused on young people who became sick or died of this disease, often directly stating that everyone is at equal risk and has to take precautions. Such misinformation led to inappropriate fear within low-risk groups and also to a lack of focus on protecting high-risk groups.

If the experts and policymakers do not communicate risk accurately, then it becomes difficult to confront the pandemic in a rational manner. For instance, if a young person believes himself or herself to be at risk, he/she may withdraw from society, not go to work, not see friends, wear masks everywhere, and self-isolate. All of which can cause deep physical and psychological harm. On the other hand, the more vulnerable elders may not believe their risk to be high. As with all medical interventions, it is important to understand the risks and benefits of our interventions to control a disease, and we can only do that if we know the risks of the disease itself, something that COVID-19 communication failed to convey.

COVID-19 is a disease that is most dangerous to very specific and easily identified groups, primarily those individuals over the age of 80 and also some who are younger who suffer from obesity, diabetes, or several other chronic medical conditions. While people who are young and healthy do get sick and die of COVID-19, their risk of this virus is no worse than the risk of many other common ailments that people face every day and that don't lead to a closure of society.

Knowing the actual risk incurred by various groups can help shape a COVID-19 policy that effectively protects those most vulnerable without causing harm to those least vulnerable. However, due to poor communication by individuals and groups deemed to be experts, the age-specific risk of COVID-19 has largely been buried in generalizations.

In the following BRCTs, we look at the risk of death in various age groups. We are focusing on the first six months of the crisis, since that is when many of our communication errors occurred and continue to this day. Since then, due to a higher rate of detection of the disease and due to better treatments, death rates have decreased overall. A *Forbes* article from October 2020 presents CDC data in the form of a bar graph; we have placed that data in a theater.

Even if public health concerns lead to a decision that all cases of COVID-19 should be assessed as equally dangerous (that even disease in young people can trigger surges in the elderly), in no way does it excuse our experts and news outlets from presenting risk accurately. If people understand their individual risk, it would allay their anxiety about COVID-19 and help them to engage in life, while helping to pave a public policy that is focused more on vulnerable people and less on those whose risk is minimal.

Out of 100,000 people aged 0–20 who get COVID-19, 3 will die.

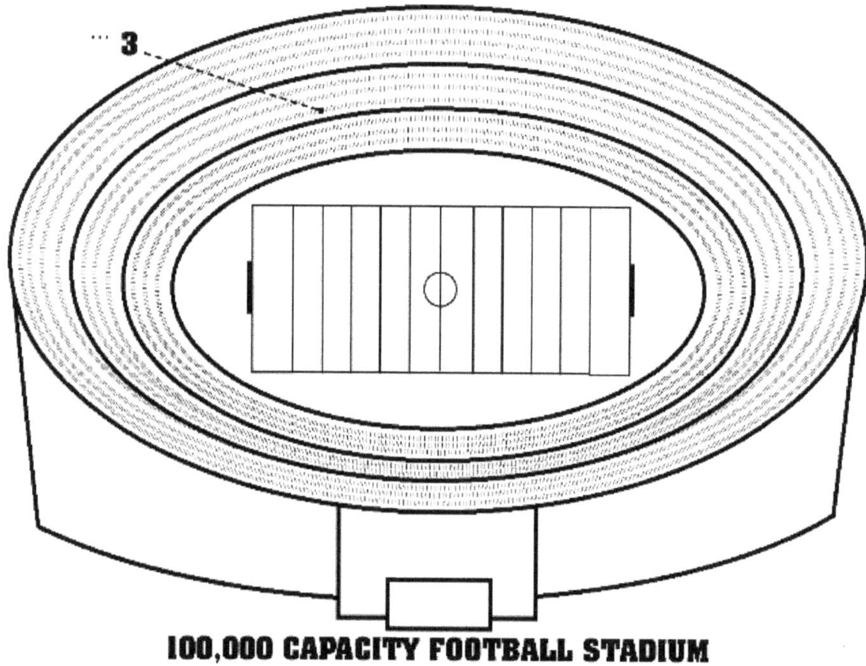

Out of 100,000 people aged 0–20, 52 will die of other causes this year.

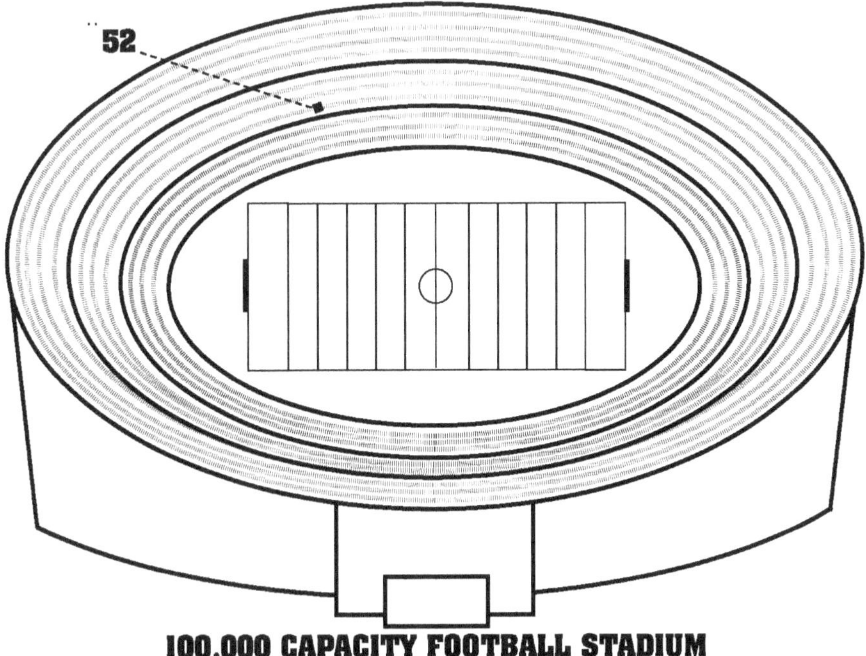

Out of 100,000 people aged 21–50 who get COVID-19, 20 will die of it.

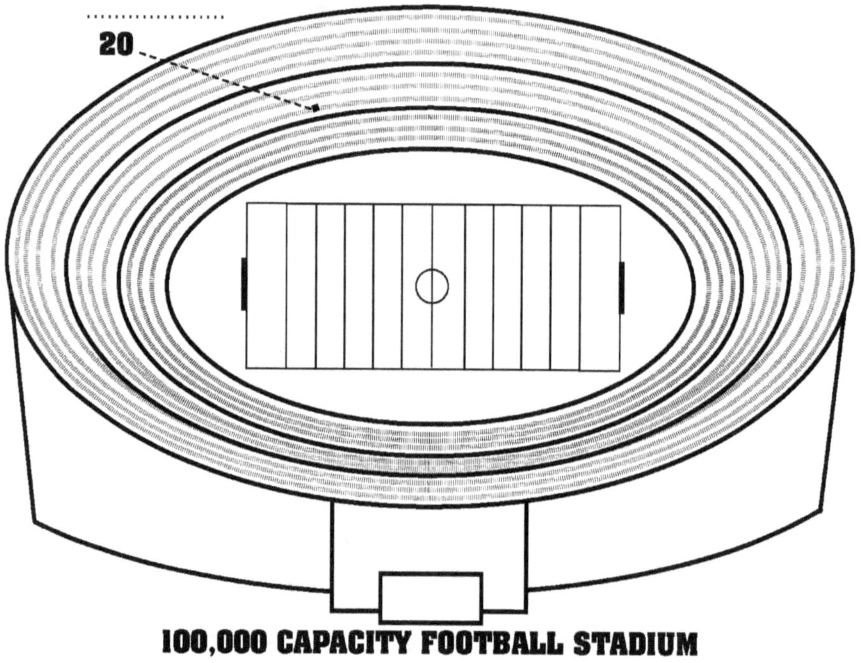

Out of 100,000 people aged 21–50, 170 will die of other causes this year.

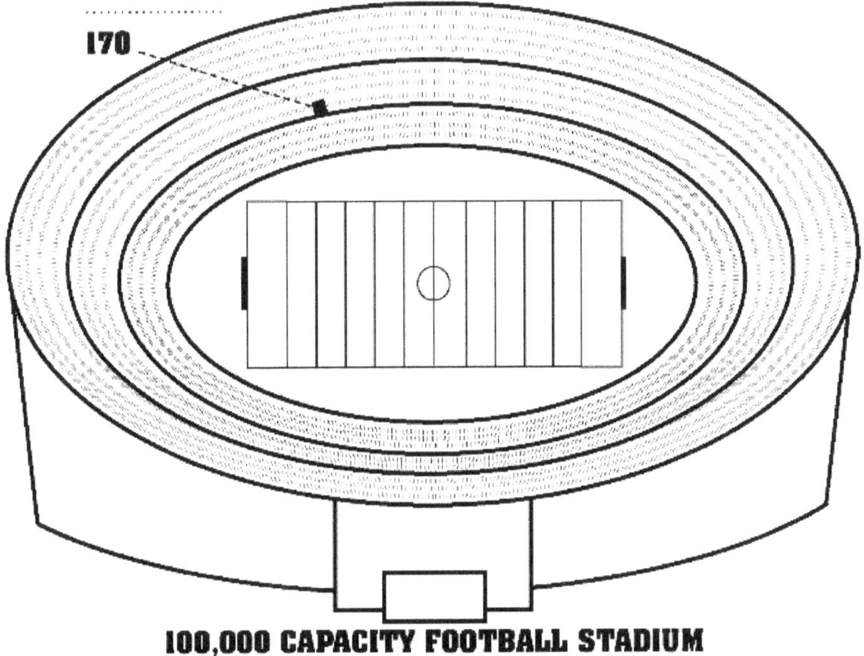

Out of 1,000 people aged 51–70 who get COVID-19, 5 will die of it.

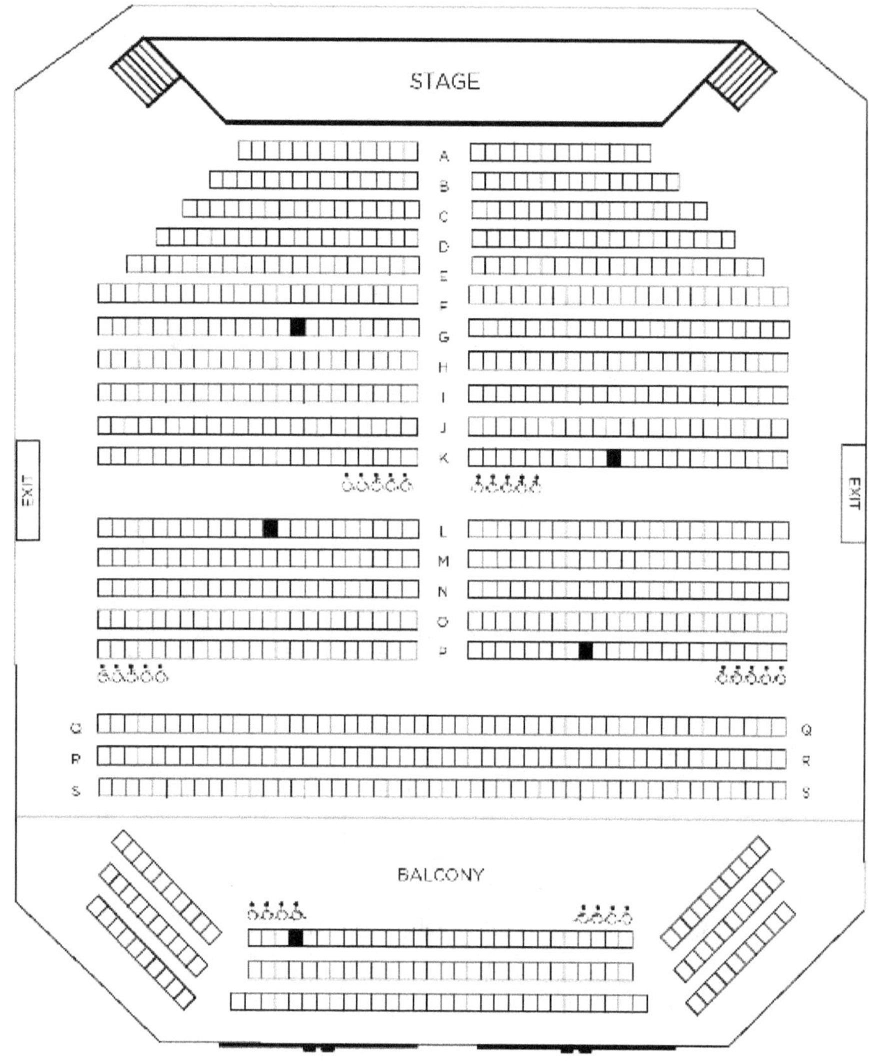

Out of 1,000 people aged 51–70, 10 will die of other causes this year.

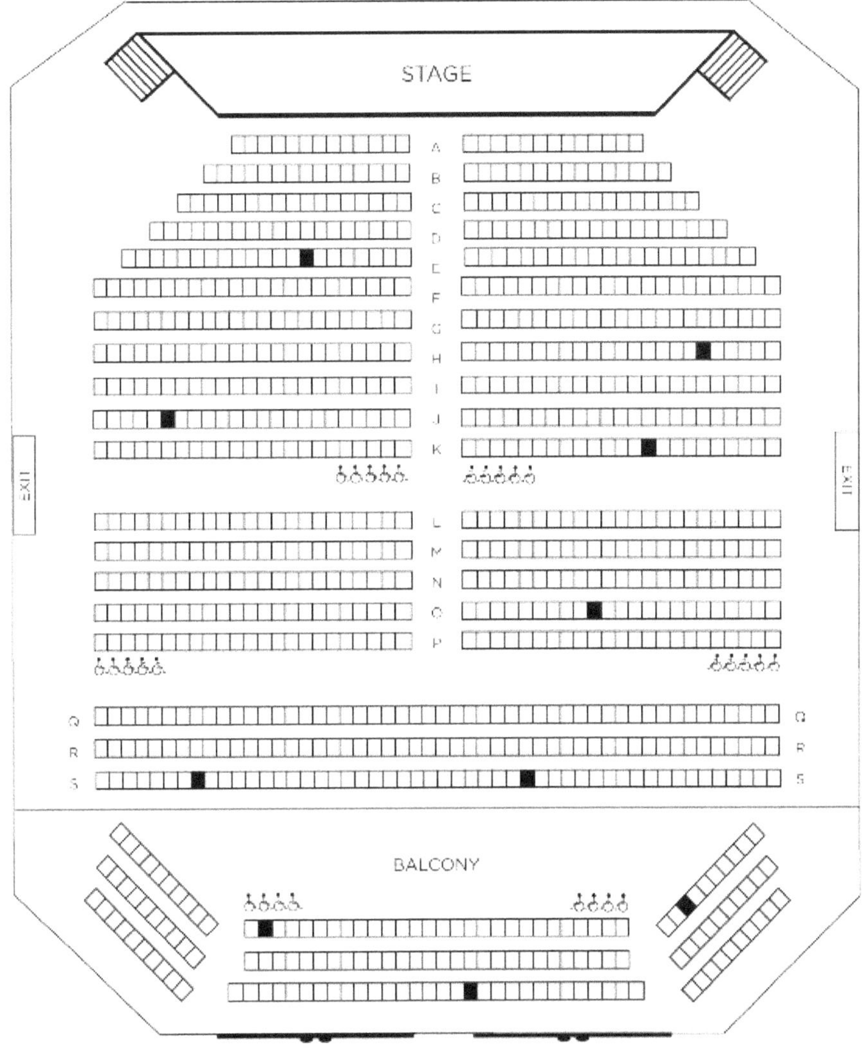

Out of 1,000 people over the age of 70 who get COVID-19, 54 will die of it.

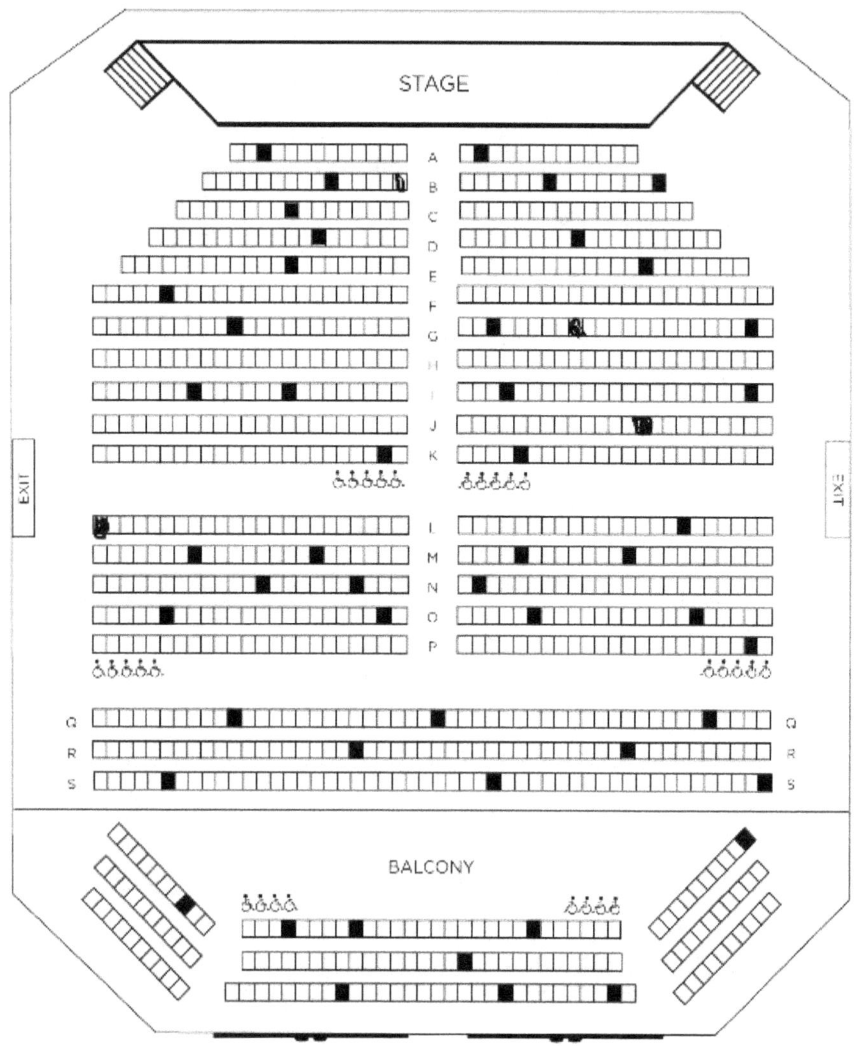

Out of 1,000 people over the age of 70, 38 will die of other causes this year.

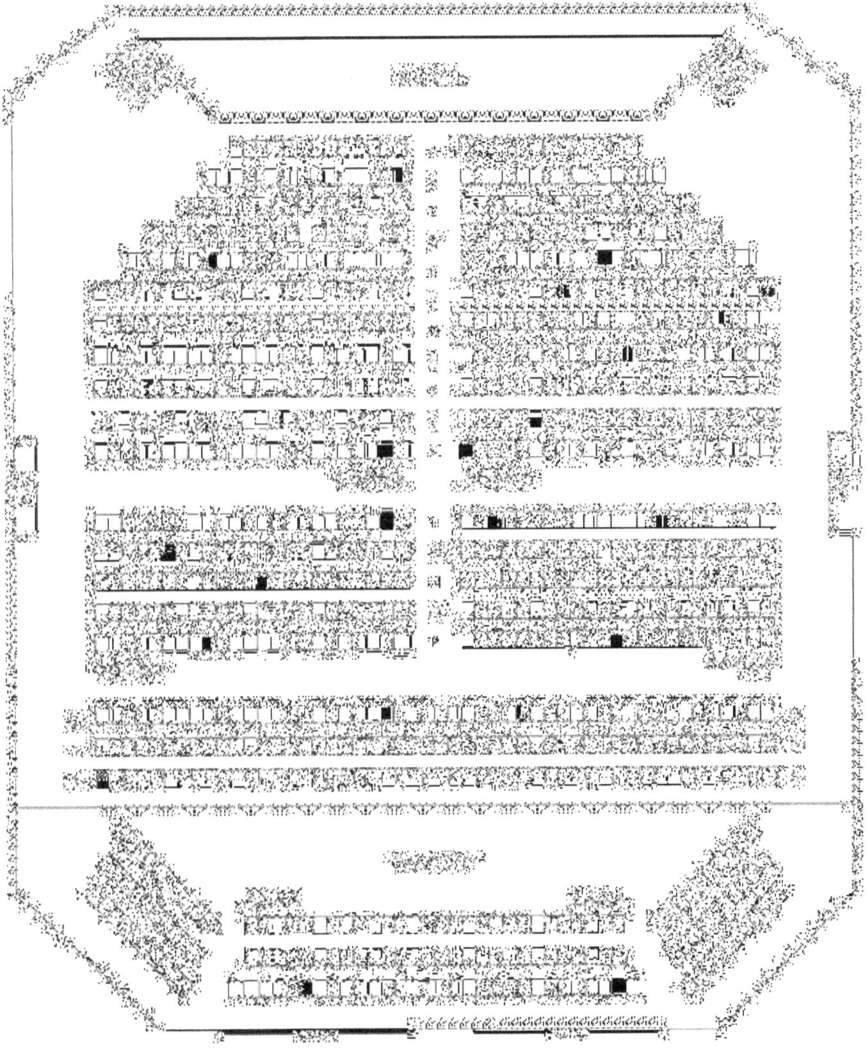

SUMMARY

To assure accurate communication regarding an individual's risk of COVID-19, compared to the risks they face every day, it is important to present that information in a clear and accurate format. Unfortunately, the media and many experts have not always been forthright. Even if public health policy attempts to reduce the overall disease burden in society, it is clear from the BRCTs that some groups have a very low risk of dying of COVID-19 compared to the risks they face every day, and any individual and policy decisions should be made with this information made clear and transparent to everyone.

- While in school-age children there is a measurable risk of death and illness with COVID-19, this risk is far lower than the risks faced every day by that demographic group.
- As age increases, so does the risk of death from COVID-19 and from other causes. Only when age is over 70 does the risk of dying of COVID-19 surpass that of risks we face and accept every day.
- A public policy discussion that acknowledges the dramatic departure of risk between ages could have more effectively pro-tected those at higher risk and, at the same time, lessened fear and restrictions among those at lower risk. What happened was a consequence of poor communication.
- While individual instances of death in low-risk populations can be identified and broadcast by media outlets and by experts, this is true of all illnesses and risks. The fact is that about a thousand kids and young adults die of auto accidents every year, and if we broadcast those deaths on the news without accurately showing how low that risk is overall, we may well prevent all kids and young adults from being in cars and buses. That is why it is important to not only show the risk in an accurate way but to compare that risk to other risks we readily accept.
- There are very real, measurable, and important consequences of isolating and quarantining people for a year, something we will

describe in a following chapter. Therefore, knowing the risk of dying of COVID-19 in each demographic group, disseminating that information accurately and clearly, and then basing policy decisions on both individual risk and the risk of a prolonged quarantine will help to lessen both the danger of the disease and of the cure.

* Any communication that obscures the truth is, by definition, not scientific and can lead to poor decisions by both individuals and by policymakers. This has certainly been the case with COVID-19, where accurate communication could have led to better outcomes and less fear.

CHAPTER 2

How safe would it be to open schools and colleges?

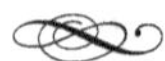

As INFORMATION ABOUT THE SAFETY of opening schools in the wake of the COVID-19 pandemic becomes available, more states and nations are enabling children to attend both primary schools and colleges. There are two concerns about allowing schools to open. First, there is the danger to students and teachers. As we have shown, children and young adults have a very low risk of dying from COVID-19, far lower than risks that they face every day and which do not lead to school closings. In fact, a flu epidemic that killed 60,000–80,000 Americans in 2017, and did impact young people far more than COVID-19, led to no school closures and very little press attention. This was considered an acceptable risk.

The second reason for containing schools is the fear of the spread of the virus from students to the community at large. This has been looked at by several US and European studies, the largest of which was in <u>France</u>, and which showed no significant illness among kids infected with COVID-19, and no substantial spread of disease from students to teachers or to the community in general. In nations that have allowed schools to remain open, there has been no surge of cases that could be linked to those schools.

Again, it is important to assess both the risk and the benefit of any policy and to communicate those risks and benefits clearly. The benefit of closing schools would be to protect students from the virus and to reduce the spread of disease from schools to the community. As we noted, none of these benefits has been shown to be found. What is the risk of closing schools?

This is much more complex, as this aspect has been poorly studied, but certainly, it has to be considered when we convolute school closures. Students are deprived of a crucial academic, social, athletic, and developmental experience. Schools, especially colleges and private schools, are deprived of income.

Measuring these deleterious consequences of school closures is crucial if we are to determine if this is good policy. Were there more suicides, more depression, and more domestic violence from closing schools? Did students lose opportunities that will impact them in both the short and the long term? Will colleges have to close? We must understand and communicate these risks of our treatment and juxtapose them with the benefits of our treatment to better understand the full impact of our COVID-19 policies, which in this case is the generalized closure of schools.

Throughout the pandemic, discussions about school closures were replete with misinformation and were confusing. To understand the risks of COVID-19 to students, and to understand which policies best reduce those risks without causing more harm, we have to compare the risk of COVID-19 to the risks faced every day and yet do not lead to school closings.

While COVID-19 communication has neglected this, we have done it in our BRCTs. As noted, it would be relevant to also construct BRCTs that demonstrate the harmful impact of school closings on students, but much of that information is currently lacking. To fully understand the impact of this treatment policy, we will need to be more open about the damaging effects of school closings as more information becomes available.

Also, though the CDC offers guidance about how to open schools safely, they have been less than forthright in their advice. They state that mask use is necessary, but they offer no data that masks worn by students lower individual risk or the risk of transmission and also ignore the possible negative effect of prolonged mask use on students, which we will explore in a later chapter.

They also state that students must be separated by six feet, sometimes changing it to three feet, without providing any scientific documentation about either. Again, accurate communication is crucial for good policy.

Out of 100,000 student-age kids and young adults who get COVID-19, 5 will die of it.

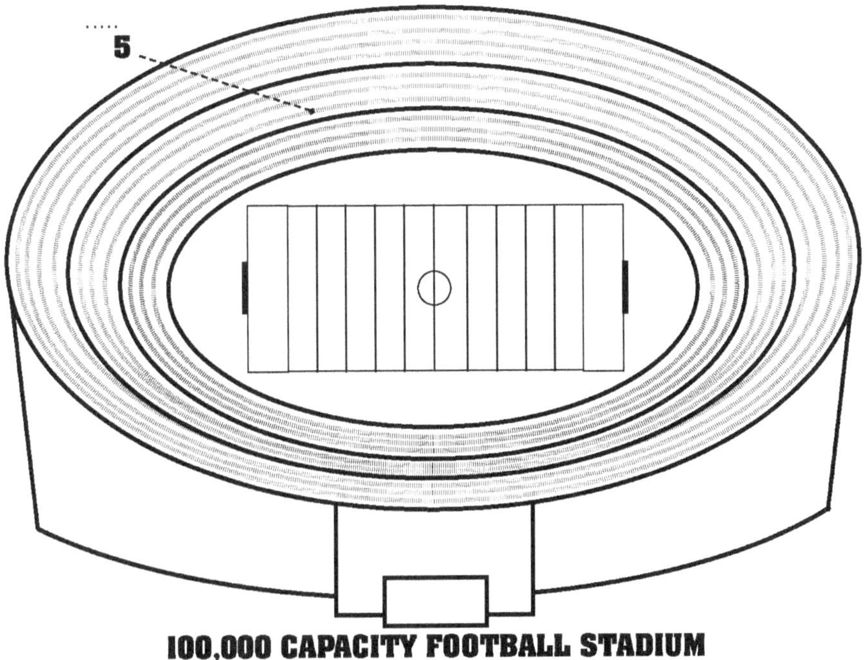

100,000 CAPACITY FOOTBALL STADIUM

Out of 100,000 college students, 11 die of accidents every year.

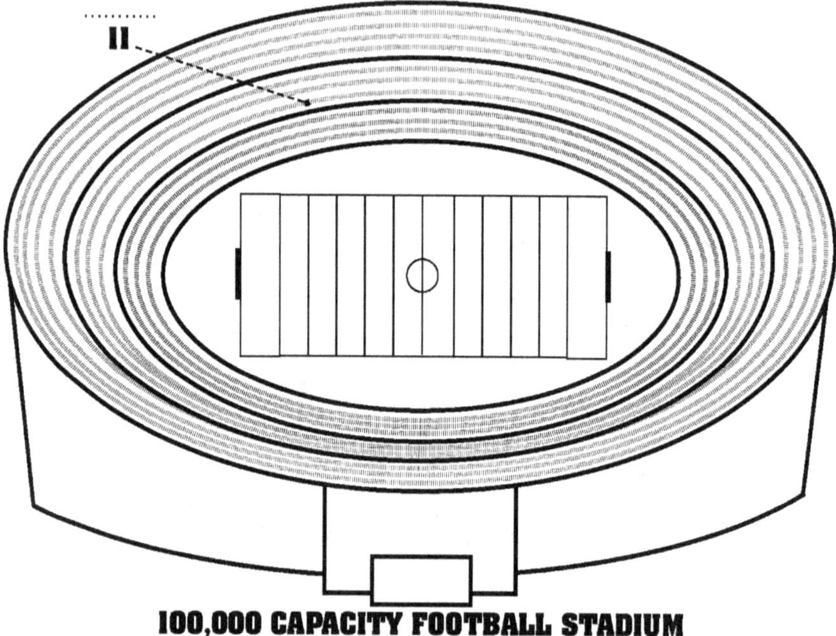

Out of 100,000 college students, on an average, 6 die of suicide every year.

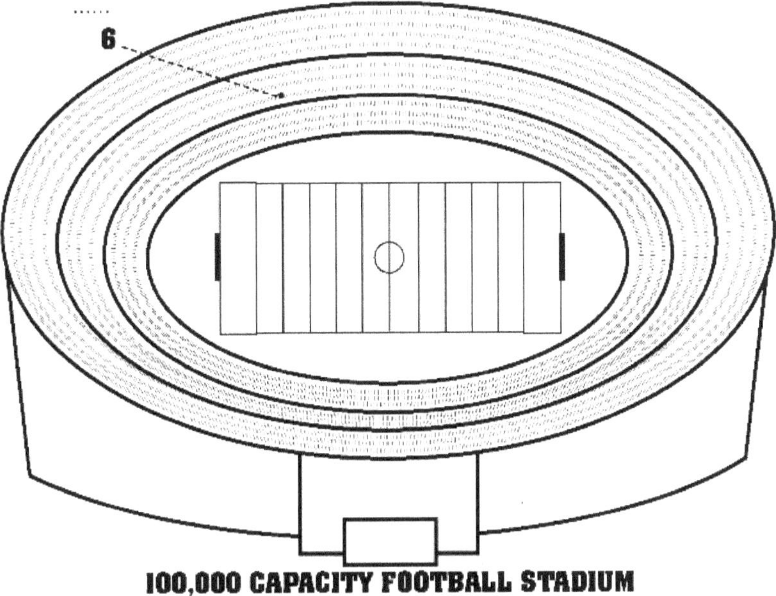

Out of 100,000 college-aged kids in 2017, 50 died of influenza in 2017.

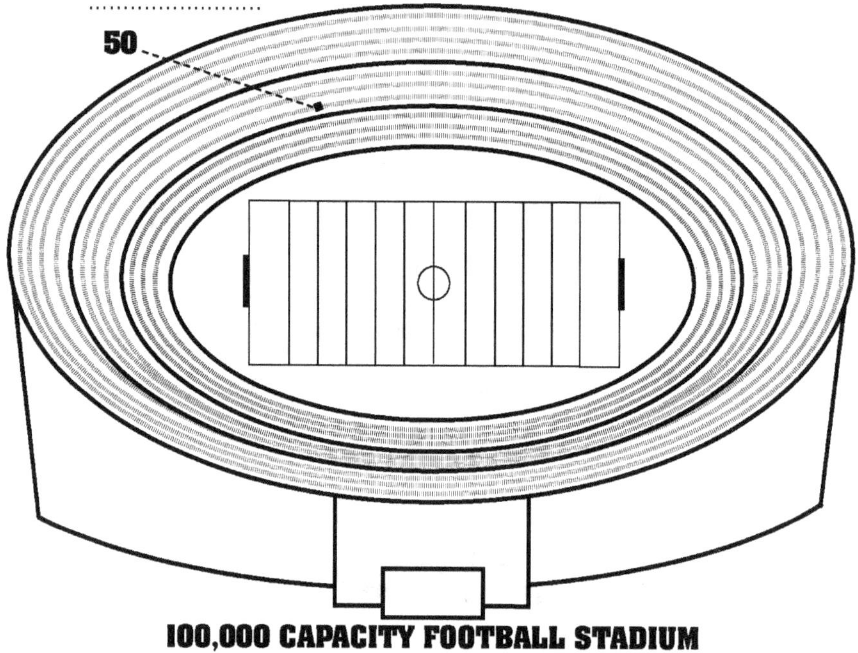

Out of 1,000 students, we are not sure how many will be harmed by closing school.

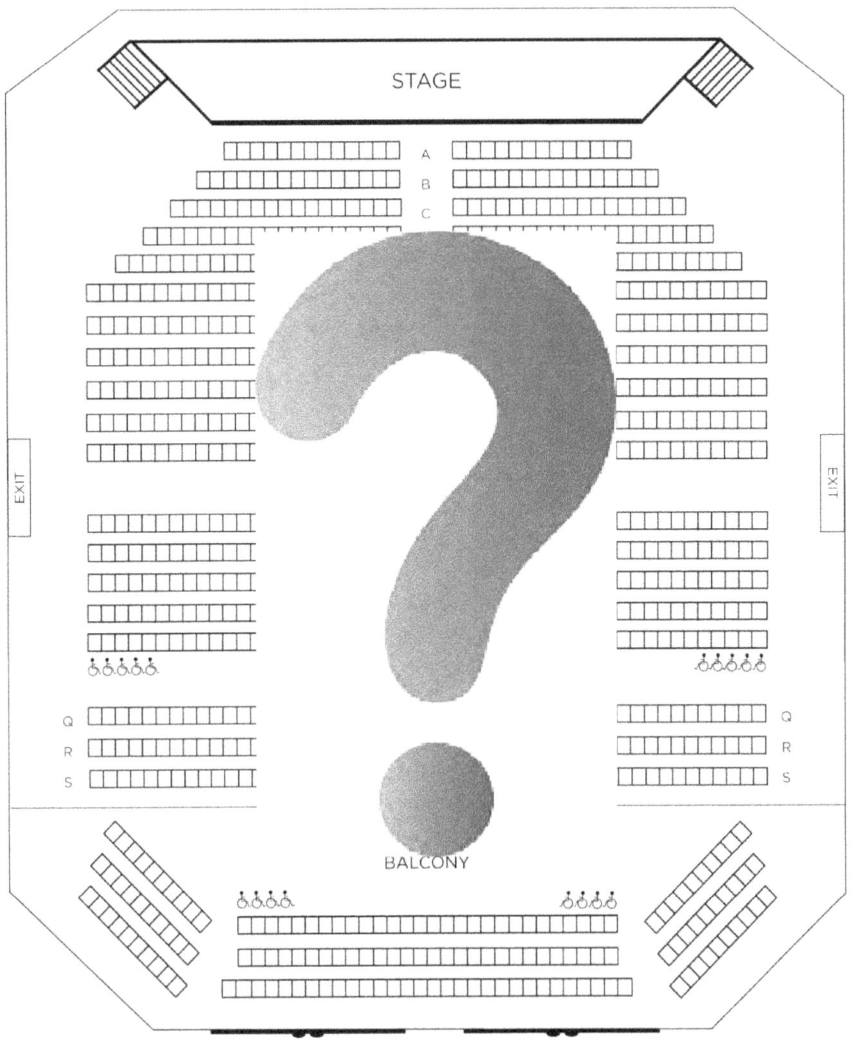

Out of 1,000 people, we are not sure if any death by COVID-19 has been prevented by closing all schools.

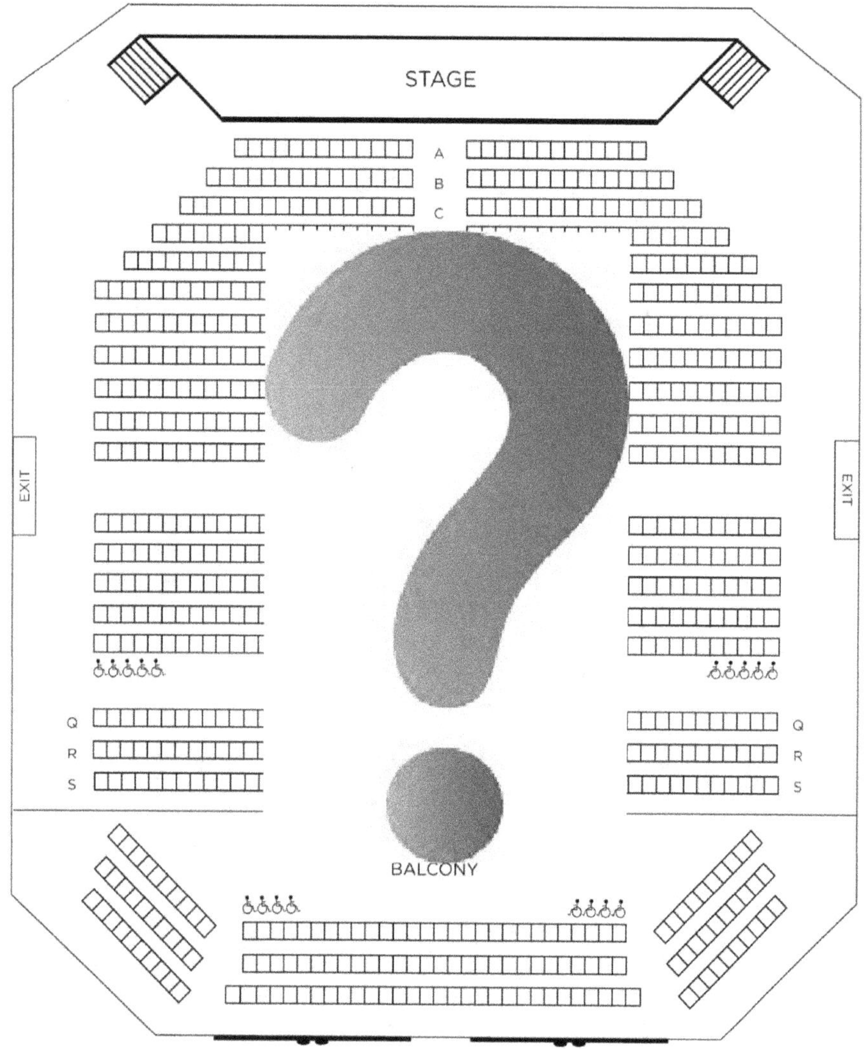

Summary

Given the low risk to students in both secondary schools and colleges from COVID-19 and the lack of evidence that opening schools will trigger a surge of COVID-19 in the community in general, the communication about school closings has been flawed and misleading, potentially raising people's fears inappropriately and leading to policy decisions based on inaccurate data.

The detrimental impact of school closings on students, communities, and institutions is rarely discussed by the media and COVID-19 experts. When it is discussed, the impact is seen as being necessary or is ascribed to COVID-19 itself. It is crucial that when we determine the impact of our treatment of a disease (in this case, the treatment is school closings), we do not convolute the adverse effects of the treatment with that of the disease. COVID-19 itself has a very small effect on students; it is no worse than the risks they face on a regular basis—which society sees as acceptable risks. The policy of closing schools, and the damage and harmful effects it may or may not have caused, must be assessed as being a consequence of our treatment, not of the disease.

All treatments have benefits and risks, and to be able to assess the overall efficacy of our COVID-19 treatment we must be forthright in communicating the effects of the disease AND the treatment separately so we can better understand what will be the best policy, moving forward. This axiom is true of all medical interventions, and it is best relayed through BRCTs. The following are several salient points:

- The risk of students dying or becoming sick from COVID-19 is lower than the risks they face every day and which do not lead to school closures.
- While less than 100 students died of COVID-19 in the first six months of the pandemic, approximately 1,000 college-aged students died of influenza in 2017, which led to no closures. Every year, just among college students, 2,000 die of car accidents, 1,000 of suicide, and 100 of homicide. There are approximately

700 alcohol-related deaths every year among college students. Just this year, pneumonia killed far more students than did COVID-19, and every year students die of infectious diseases in numbers that far exceed that of COVID-19 deaths, and yet none of these deaths have led to school closures.

* There is no evidence that opening schools will lead to dangerous surges in society.

* It is important to know whether school closings have had a measurable detrimental impact on students so we can compare the risks of our treatment with the risks of the disease itself. Were there more suicides, more domestic violence, more alcohol-related injuries, and more depression? Can we measure how much students suffered from being deprived of social interaction, athletics, school activities, in-person classes, graduations, internships, and so much else? Currently, we have a BRCT with a ? to show this, but to understand the true effect of our COVID-19 policy, we must calculate the harm incurred by our treatment of the disease in a concrete way that can be put into a BRCT.

* It is important also to calculate the economic impact of school closures on institutions, employees of those institutions, community businesses that are dependent on schools for their business, etc. All of this can and must be put into a BRCT.

* As mentioned, it is neither accurate nor constructive to ascribe the detrimental effects of school closings to COVID-19 itself. COVID-19 did not close schools; our treatment of COVID-19 did, and thus must we weigh the risks and benefits of that treatment and compare it with the risk of COVID-19 to students and society had we allowed schools to open.

* It is similarly not accurate or constructive to list necessary protective measures that must be used in schools, from masks and distancing, without ascertaining their benefits and risks.

CHAPTER 3

Long-term care, the focus of infection; how well did we do?

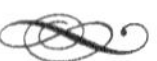

IF YOUNG PEOPLE WHO ATTEND schools are at very low risk from COVID-19, frail elders are at the highest risk. Many frail elders live in long-term care, whether in nursing homes or in assisted living residences, and nationally the deaths from COVID-19 in such institutions represent about 40 percent of all deaths. Worldwide such deaths constitute almost 70 percent of all deaths.

While COVID-19 communication has to some extent acknowledged the disproportionate risk of COVID-19 to residents of long-term care, it has not been transparent about the extent of that risk compared to the population as a whole, or how well our measures to mitigate that risk have helped and harmed residents of long-term care.

Long-term care institutions offer us a window into how well our measures to curb COVID-19 work in a setting in which the infection is most harmful. In one sense, because these are closed institutions, it is easy to assure compliance with policies designed to protect residents.

From the start of the pandemic, long-term care facilities required and enforced universal mask use, social isolation, screening of employees, isolation of infected individuals with contact tracking, limitation of visitation, and often even more extreme measures such as forcing elders to remain in their rooms and the use of shields and gowns by all staff.

Thus, assessing how we did in long-term care facilities can reveal the benefit and risk of our measures to curb COVID-19. Unfortunately, communication about COVID-19 rarely focused on this vulnerable population and did not accurately convey the risks and benefits of our treatment attempts to curb COVID-19 deaths among them. ***The results of this often misleading and neglectful communication have been catastrophic.***

Our BRCTs show that the risk of death due to COVID-19 is higher among long-term care residents than among people who live in the community. Overall, the risk of dying of COVID-19 in long-term care among those infected with the virus is 85/1,000, while the average risk to people not in long-term care is 1/2,000. This is a striking difference, and, if accurately conveyed, could have led to policies that focused on long-term care, rather than on policies that precipitated total society shutdowns.

While experts and policymakers accurately note that surges within communities often correspond to surges in long-term care (mostly because workers in long-term care live in the community and thus bring in the virus), they have not demonstrated that community quarantines reduce that risk, although in their communication they assume that it has.

As nursing home deaths mounted despite societal quarantines, communication about this did not reflect a growing reality that shutting down society was not keeping the virus out of our long-term care facilities or reducing deaths there. A BRCT with a "**?**" shows that such a policy has uncertain benefits.

Similarly, the universal use of personal protective equipment (**PPE**) and masks, as well as strict quarantine and tracking policies within facilities, continues to be touted as the best way to mitigate the impact of viral spread in long-term care. This is again a communication failure.

The nearly 200,000 residents of long-term care who died from COVID-19 were infected by the virus despite a strict quarantine within facilities, universal masking by all employees, no family visits, and employee screening. Continual statements that masks and quarantines are effective in long-term care, despite clear and compelling evidence that they are not, have led to continuing of policies that likely have not reduced the deaths among this most vulnerable population.

In addition, communication has failed to assess the detrimental effects of a prolonged quarantine on the health, psychological state, and longevity of elders who have been locked up now for over a year. To understand the efficacy of our treatment strategy we must look at both its risks and benefits, and in long-term care, we looked at neither. ***This communication failure has caused significant death and disability from the disease and the treatment, something that we will have to better assess once we look at the data.***

Out of 1,000 long-term-care residents who get COVID-19, 85 will die from it.

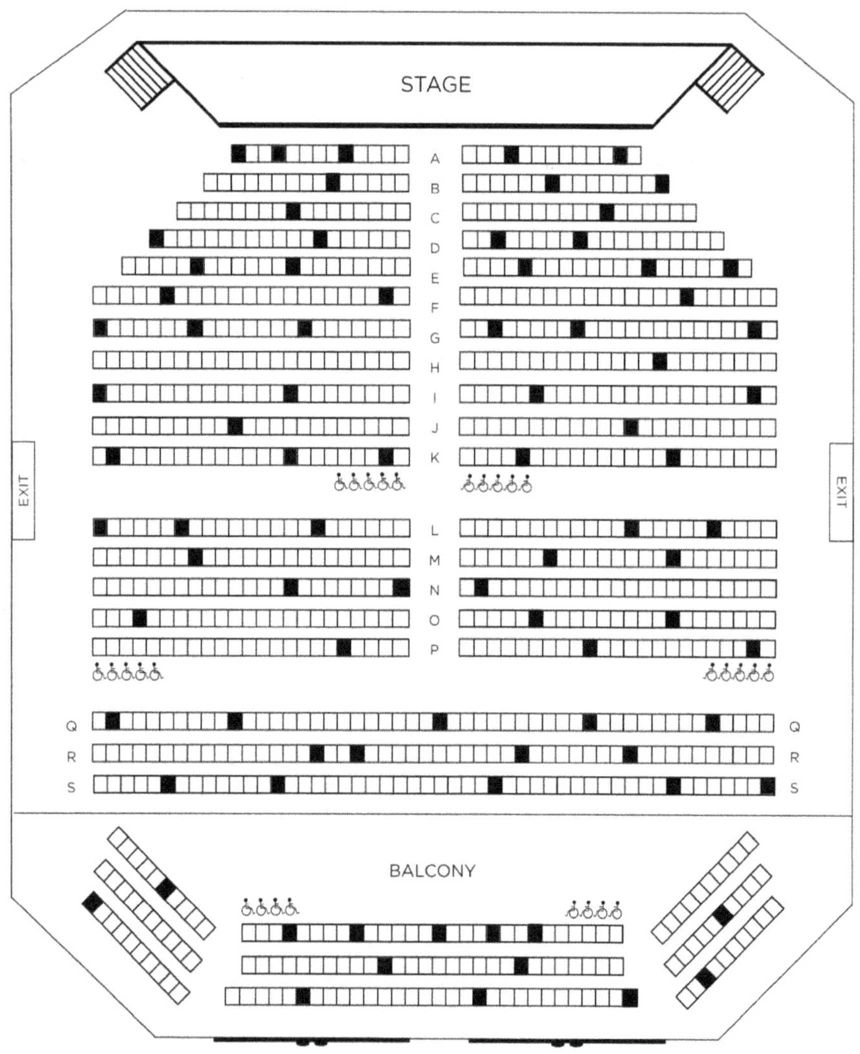

Out of 2,000 people not in long-term care and who do not live in long-term care and get COVID-19, one will die from it.

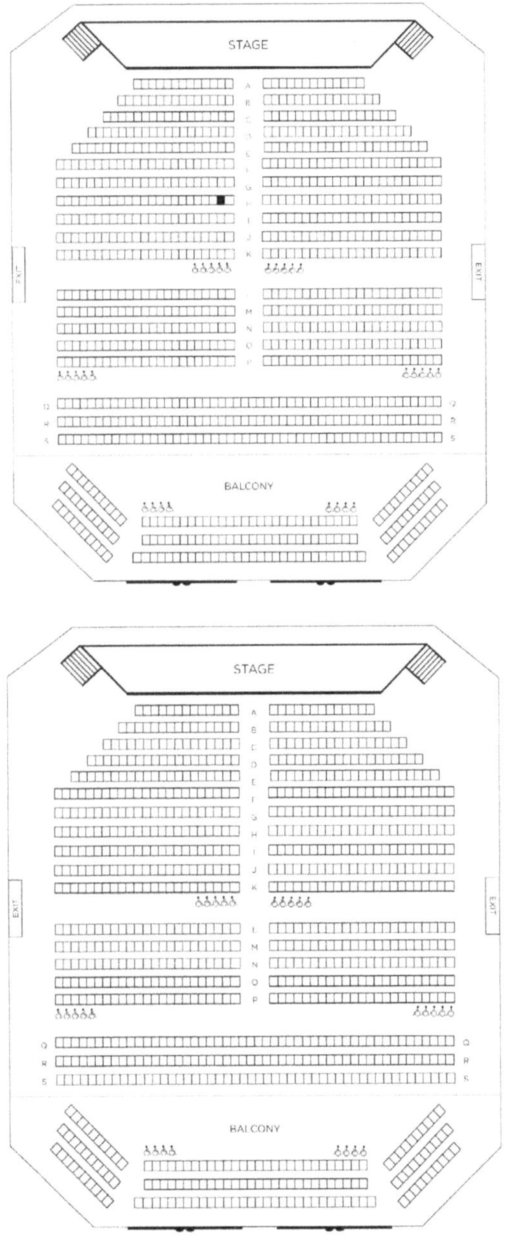

Out of 1,000 people who get influenza in an average year, 1 will die from it.

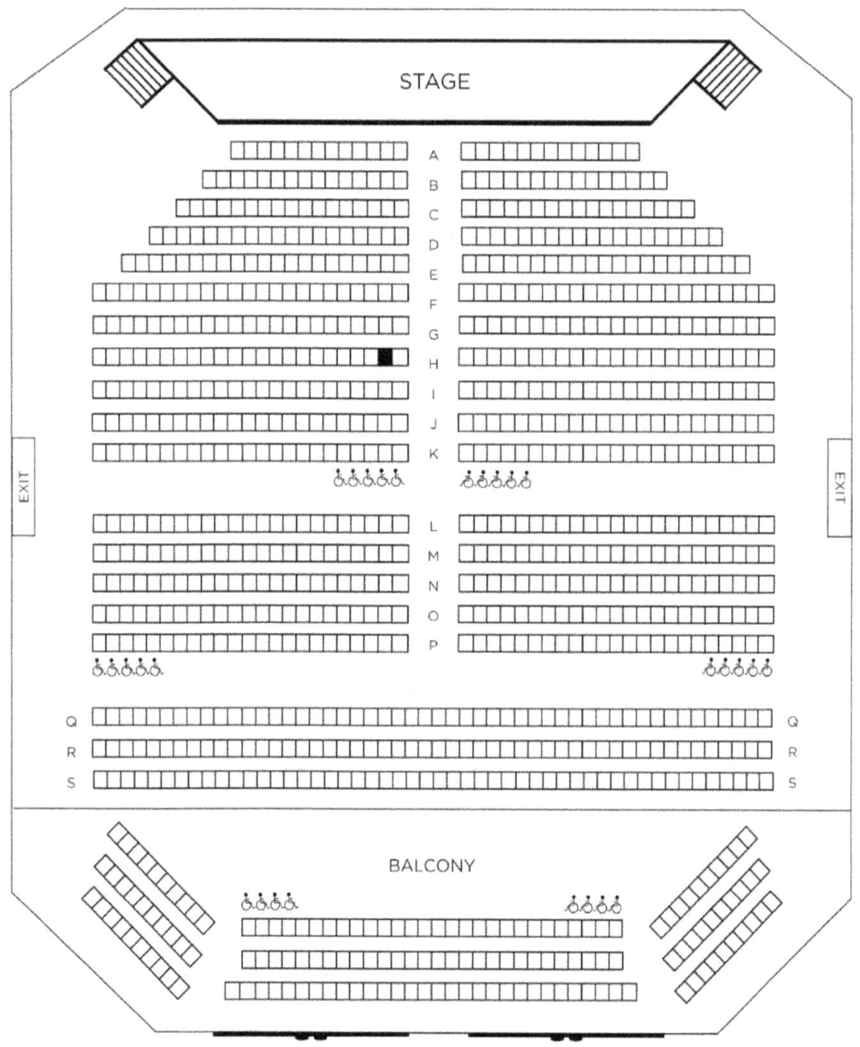

Out of 1,000 nursing homes that enforce universal mask use and strict quarantines, we do not have any evidence that any lives will be saved.

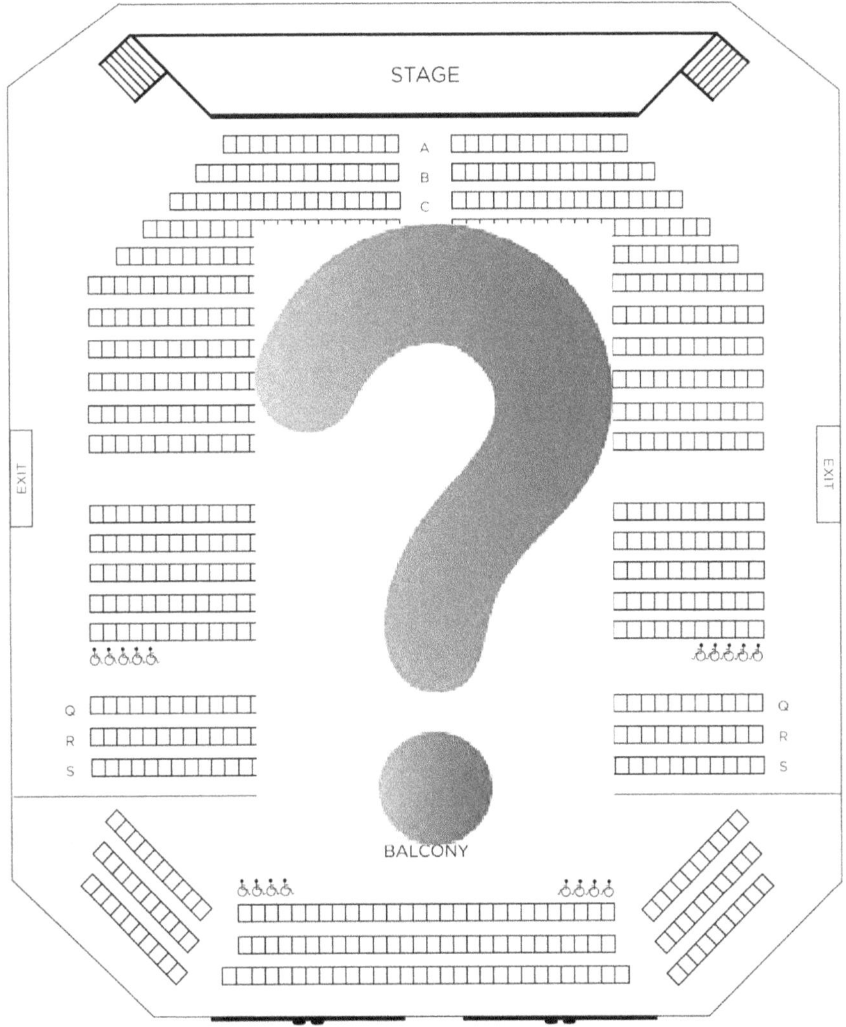

Out of 1,000 long-term care residents, there is no evidence that any lives will be saved by closing down society

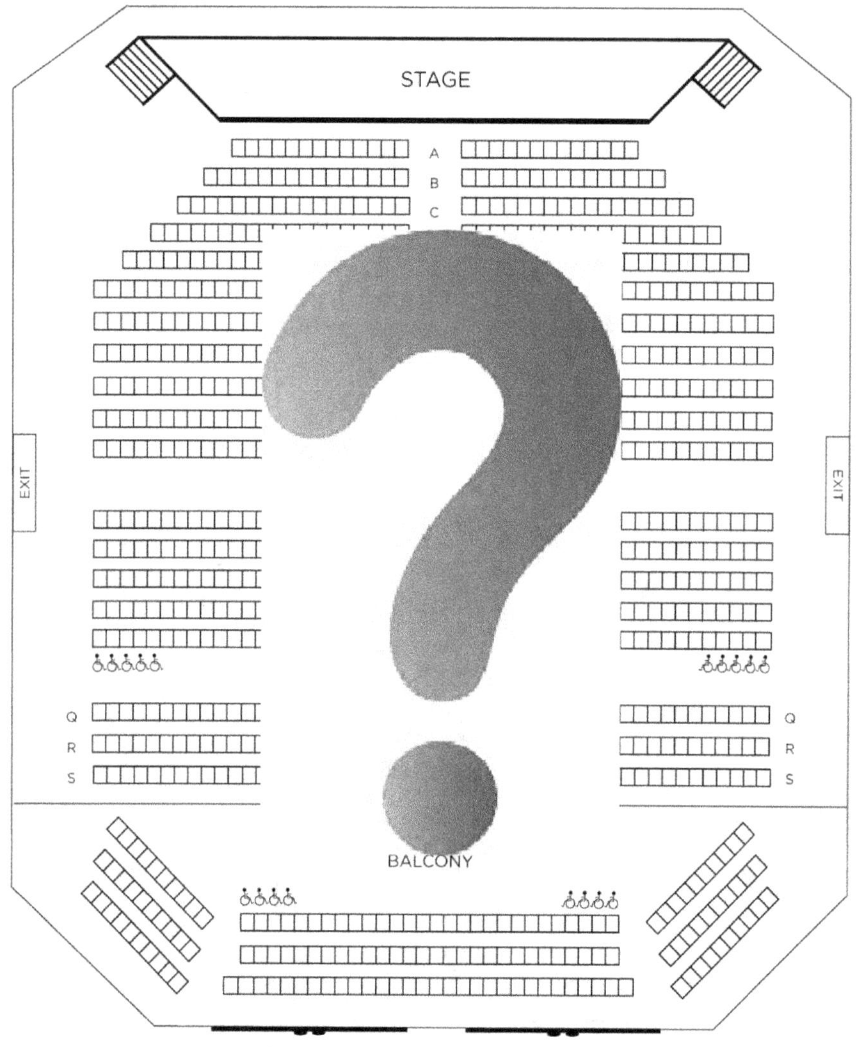

Out of 1,000 long-term care residents subjected to a prolonged quar-antine, we are unsure how many will suffer mental and physical conse-quences or death.

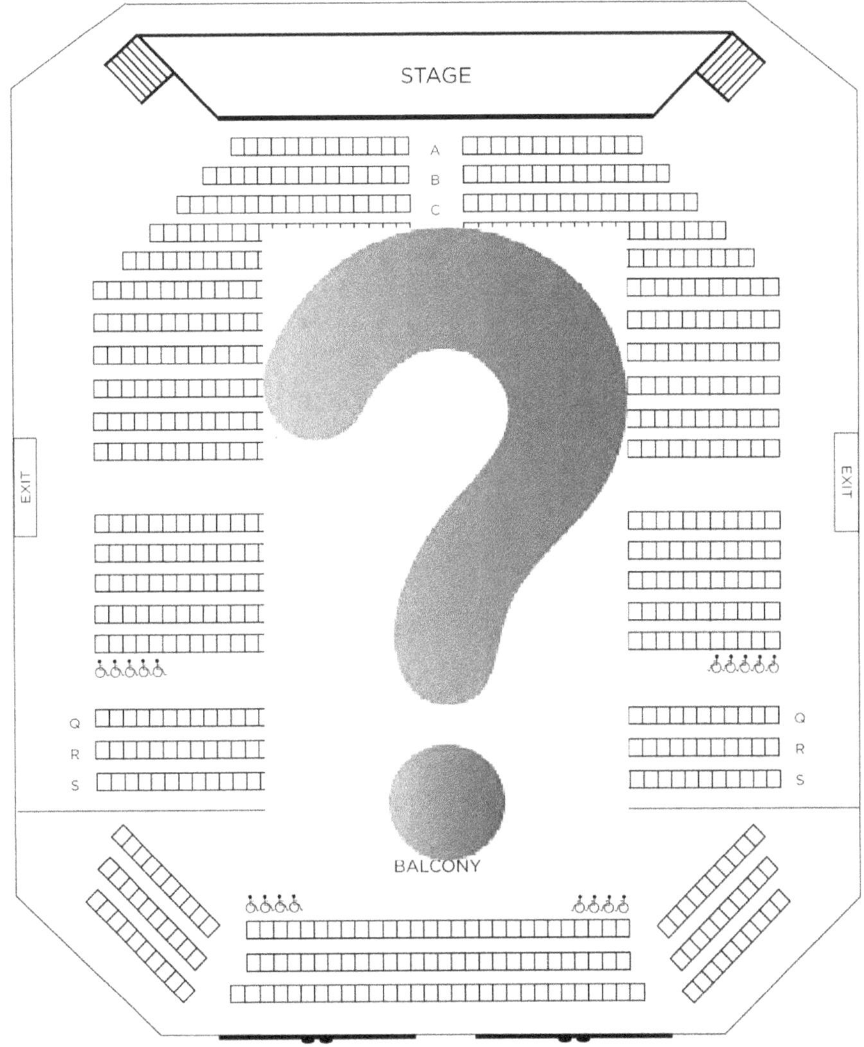

SUMMARY

Both in this country and worldwide, nursing home deaths from COVID-19 have been far higher than that of the population in general. Had communication about COVID-19 focused on this center of infection and accurately conveyed the sharp divide between long-term care residents and the rest of society in terms of COVID-19 risk, then perhaps policy decisions that focused on long-term care would have been more effective.

Instead, long-term care utilized treatments—social isolation, universal masking, limited visitation—that had no proven benefit, that likely did not reduce deaths, and that may have harmed vulnerable elders. Communication about these measures did not focus on their uncertainty regarding both benefit and risk, leading to ineffective and likely detrimental measures as our mainstay of treatment.

Similarly, communication often stated that by shutting down society—closing schools, restricting assembly and travel, closing businesses, mandating mask use everywhere—we would reduce death in long-term care. This too has no evidence of efficacy and may have led to more harm than good. Communication must be honest and clear regarding who is most vulnerable to COVID-19, the risks and benefits of our treatments to protect these people, and how we can alter our treatment to provide the most benefit and least risk. By all measures, COVID-19 communication in this arena failed, leading to disastrous consequences. Following are some salient points:

* The number of deaths among long-term care residents far exceeds that among the general population. In long-term care, 53/1,000 infected people die, compared to 1/2,000 of all those not in long-term care. Because our COVID-19 communication did not adequately emphasize the disproportionate risk among residents of long-term care, often implying that risk is ubiquitous among all demographics, we as a society did not focus on that population in our treatment strategy.

* There is no evidence that shutting down society in any way reduces the death rate in long-term care, even though there is a correlation between society surges and surges in long-term care.

* Policies within long-term care facilities, such as universal masking and strict social isolation, did not prevent COVID-19 from entering these facilities and causing significant death, despite communication from experts and policymakers that implied that they were effective. In fact, those treatments are still used without any discussion about their lack of benefit.

* Universal masking and prolonged social isolation could have significant detrimental effects in long-term care, leading to depression, dementia, falls, weakness, and death. It is important to determine the risk of our treatment and to compare that to the benefit when we ascertain whether such treatment should continue. We did not (and continue not to) do that, triggering misleading communication that suggests the necessity and efficacy of current treatment measures despite a paucity of evidence to support these claims, while neglecting any focus on the possible detrimental effects of these measures.

* It has been suggested that excess deaths and disability among residents in long-term care are from COVID-19, whereas, it is likely that they derive from our attempt to treat and control COVID-19, a distinction crucial to make if we are to best understand optimal treatment strategies. Currently, the extent of such treatment-related death and disability has not been calculated, but it will be crucial to do that and compare it to COVID-19 deaths.

CHAPTER 4

Universal masking—the danger of relying on communication from experts and not on evidence

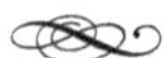

NOTHING MORE VISIBLY DEMONSTRATES OUR attempts to curb the spread and impact of COVID-19 than the prolific use of masks. Society is divided about how much masks help, even as experts continue to declare unequivocally that they are both necessary and effective in reducing death from and spread of this virus. Communication about masking has been confusing and often erroneous.

When an "expert" makes a claim about the benefit, or lack of benefit, of mask use, does that excuse the expert from buttressing his or her claim with clear and accurate evidence? When it came to masks, those who trumpeted the benefit and need of universal masking did so without any evidence to back their claims and without any concern about potential detrimental effects of prolonged mask use, leading to an assumption among the media and policymakers that the benefit of mask use was an unassailable axiom.

The value of a BRCT is demonstrated in its usefulness to assess masks in the context of their benefit and harm, especially when there is uncertainty about their efficacy. When experts, the media, and policymakers make a claim without providing evidence of benefit and risk, they are engaging in a communication failure that could lead to adverse consequences. Without evidence as to the risks and benefits of masking, it is difficult to know if masks have any value, if they are harmful to some groups or in some settings, which masks may be effective, when they should be worn, and when they may cause more harm than good. **Thus, because of flawed communication in which experts made claims in the absence of demonstrating the scientific basis of their assertions, masks have become more a symbol than a proven treatment, and it is difficult to know if they are useful or harmful.**

Before COVID-19 hit our shores, many studies had been conducted about the benefit and risks of the use of a mask in influenza pandemics. The consensus of all these studies was that for influenza, masks neither protected the wearer of masks nor curbed the spread of disease in society. Such studies are summarized in a <u>Cochrane report</u>.

After COVID-19 arrived, a WHO review of observational studies suggested that the use of primarily N95 masks in two high-risk areas—homes with a known infected person, and hospitals with multiple COVID-19 patients—could decrease transmission, without any evidence in reduction of death. This led the CDC and WHO, as well as many experts, to declare the need for universal masking, even though the studies they cited (and which they did not accurately explain) looked only at two high-risk arenas and did not demonstrate significant benefit.

Several studies after that, including a <u>randomized trial</u>, disputed the benefit of masks in a community setting, and <u>other studies</u> found that masks are not effective in even high-risk locations. In fact, no study has demonstrated that face mask use lessens the spread of COVID-19 or protects the wearer, and our nation's experience in nursing homes—where infections and death among workers and residents are rampant despite well-enforced universal mask use—should further dissuade any expert from declaring that masks have been proven to be beneficial and are a necessary strategy to confront this disease even in this very high-risk location.

And yet, this is exactly what experts continue to say, what many states and businesses mandate, and what has become the primary mechanism in our nation to fight COVID-19, all with a complete lack of evidence of efficacy. **In this regard, masks represent a symbol of something very**

wrong with our COVID-19 communication and, indeed, with communication throughout the heath care arena: experts seem not accountable to prove what they proclaim to be fact.

In addition, as a <u>recent review</u> has demonstrated, not only have no studies demonstrated a beneficial effect of masks, but multiple smaller studies suggest that, especially with prolonged use, mask use may cause substantial harm. While it is difficult to determine the quantity of that harm sufficiently to put it in a BRCT, and to determine who is most vulnerable to it, it is something that needs to be considered when experts and policymakers insist that masks are safe and effective and mandate their use. The truth is that we simply do not know if they help in certain settings and if they harm certain groups of people. However, we do know that they are not effective in more generalized community settings and as protection against influenza in any setting. This is all shown by our BRCTs.

Communication by experts convinces us to be confident about the benefits of an intervention that may not be effective or can cause harm, which can lead to policy decisions and to personal choices that may well be deleterious to both society and to individuals. It also may, as has been true in nursing homes, persuade institutions and policymakers to mandate ineffective and possibly harmful treatments, when other more rational strategies are shelved because we are too focused on masks.

We have used a "?" in our theater to demonstrate the uncertainty of mask efficacy in high-risk settings, although growing research shows they are likely not effective in those settings. Studies in low-risk community settings have shown them not to be effective, as shown on our BRCT, even as their use is still touted as being necessary and effective. When a treatment lacks certainty as to whether it helps and whether it harms, it is crucial that any communication about that treatment clearly reveal that uncertainty. **When we know what we don't know, then we can make decisions more productively and not rely on strategies that have little scientific validity.**

Out of 1,000 people in high-risk areas such as nursing homes and hospitals, we have no evidence that any lives will be saved with universal mask use, and no evidence that lives won't be saved.

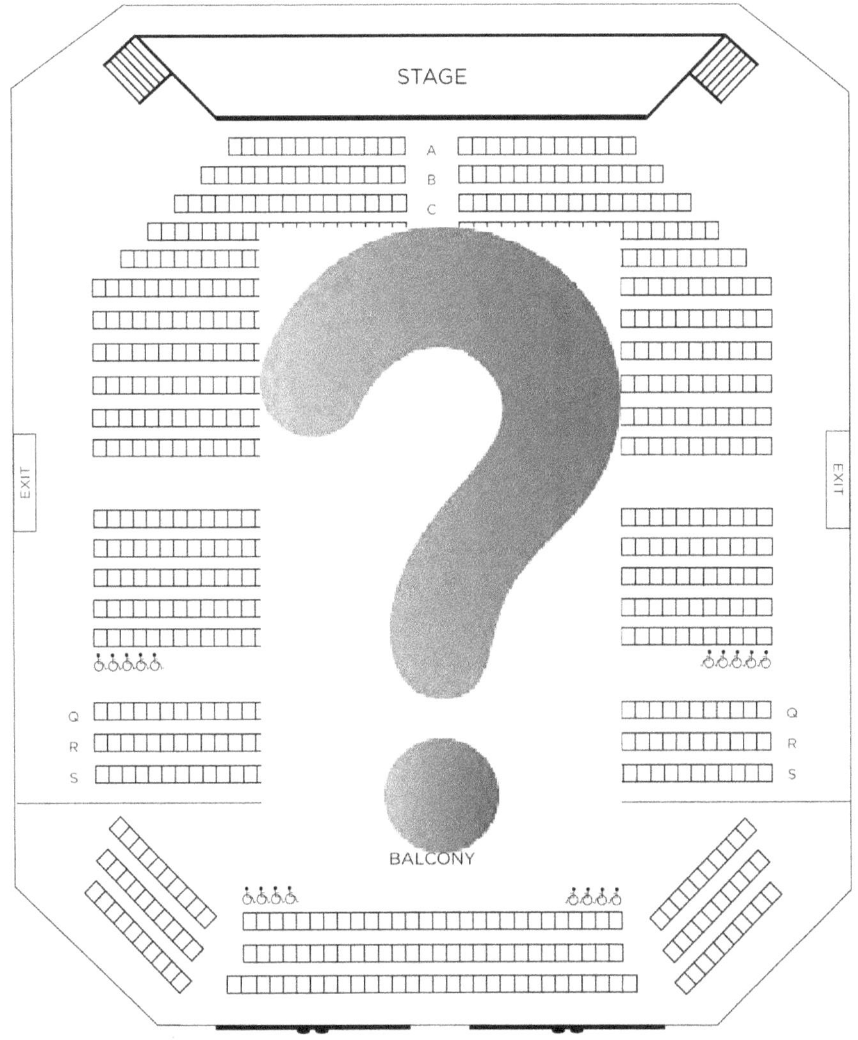

Out of 1,000 people who wear masks for a prolonged period of time, we do not know how many, if any at all, will suffer from physical and/or psychological dangers.

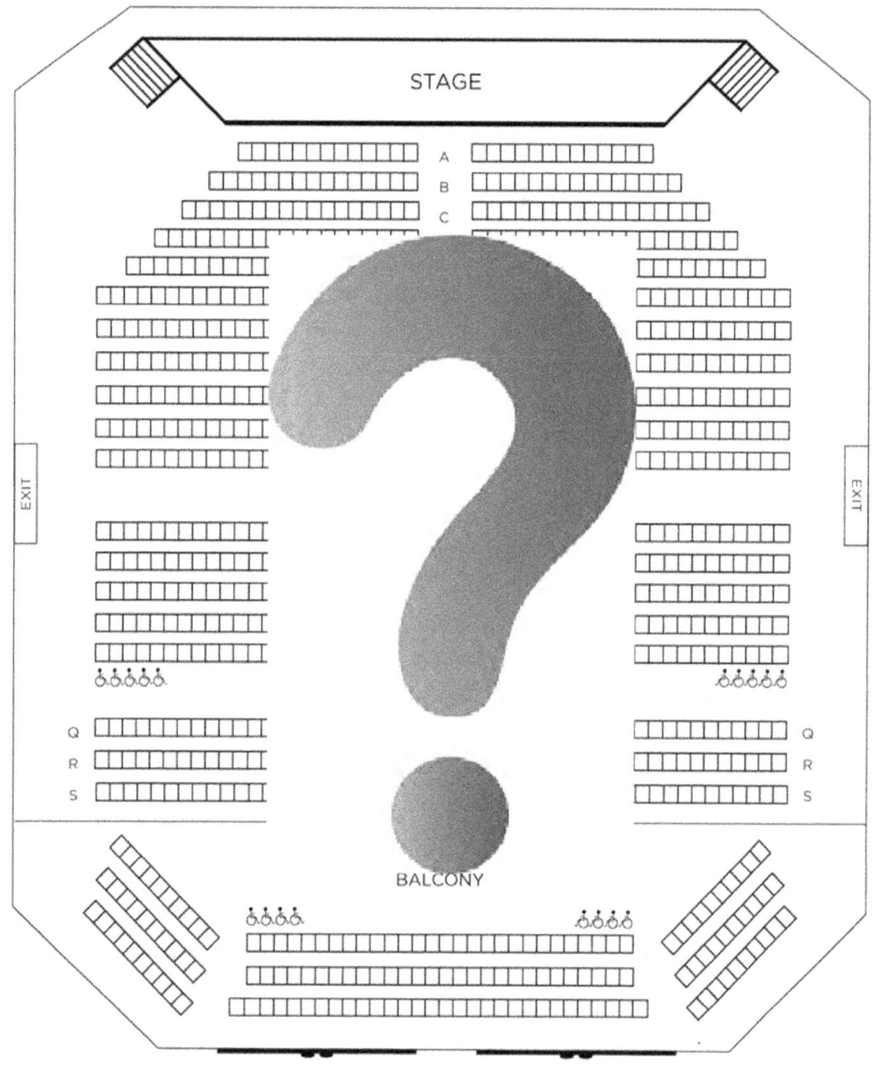

Out of 1,000 people in a community setting who wear a mask either inside or outside, data suggests that no lives will be saved. This is true of COVID-19 and influenza.

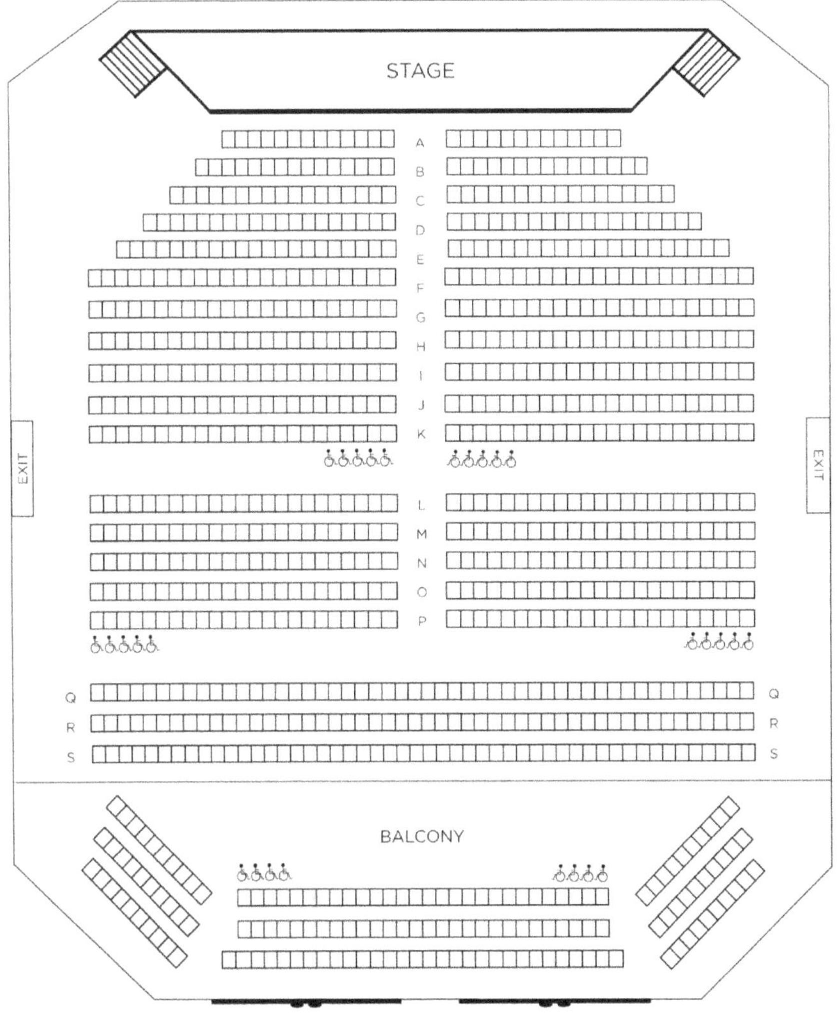

Summary

Extensive studies have been carried out on masks with regard to their protective effect in influenza, and only limited studies in terms of their potential benefit in COVID-19. While many experts have declared unequivocally that masks are essential to protect the wearer and to curb the spread of disease, such statements have no scientific backbone to support them.

Perhaps one of the most glaring deficiencies of COVID-19 communication—and one that is universal in health care generally—is the gap between what experts proclaim to be true and what we know (or don't know) to be actually true. Nothing represents this more than universal mask use, which has never been shown to protect the wearer or prevent disease spread in any setting and has been shown to be ineffective in the community setting where its use is both mandated and relied upon as the mainstay of our treatment.

In addition, few who advocate mask use even discuss the possible side effects of this treatment, which may, in fact, be substantial, or may be trivial; we simply do not know. Hence, due to poor COVID-19 communication—mostly from experts who do not feel the need to rely on scientific evidence to back up what they say, and from the media, which has not demanded such evidence—masks have become our nation's most touted weapon against COVID-19, even in the absence of any proof that they work and that they don't cause harm.

This is why communication in all realms of health care must be honest and clear, even when there is uncertainty; otherwise, we could be basing policy and personal decisions on dogma rather than science and cause more harm than good. Following are a few salient points:

* The use of masks in influenza has been well studied and shown to be ineffective. This year, where deaths from influenza have been few, many experts are tying that reduction in death to prolific mask use, a declarative statement that we know is scientifically erroneous.

- COVID-19 is similar to influenza in how it is spread, and thus many groups, including Cochrane, postulate that masks will neither protect the mask wearer from COVID-19 infection nor curb disease spread, based on data from influenza.
- We cannot be certain that masks convey no protection in high-risk environments such as nursing homes and hospitals, although data would suggest that they are not effective. More study is needed in this area.
- On the basis of randomized studies and copious observational data, we can be fairly certain that masks convey no protection in community settings. The use of masks outdoors, in stores, in restaurants, etc., which has been declared by experts as necessary, has not helped.
- We are unsure if masks are risky to the wearer, but some evidence suggests that they may be, especially with prolonged use, and especially among the young and the old, two groups who are most likely to be mandated to wear a mask.
- Other similar measures—such as plexiglass barriers, face shields, gloves, hand sanitizer, six-foot distancing, and one-way aisles in stores—have no evidence of efficacy in any setting, and some may even cause harm. Like with masks, experts declare these measures to be effective and necessary without providing any data to support their claims.
- It should be clear that all people, even those who declare themselves experts, must present data to back up their claims, and the data should be presented in a BRCT form so that it represents actual risks/benefits and can be easily understood
- When we are unsure about whether an intervention may harm or help the condition we are using it to treat, it is important to convey that uncertainty, as we have done with a ? in our BRCTs.

CHAPTER 5

The efficacy of quarantines: why we must discuss benefits AND risks of treatments

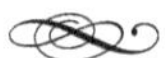

ASIDE FROM MASK USE, THE top-down mandates of social distance and quarantine have been communicated by experts as being effective and necessary to prevent deaths from and spread of COVID-19. But, despite the assuredness of such communication, and the willingness of federal and state agencies to mandate quarantines, how much do we know about the benefits and risks of this strategy?

The answer is, we don't know. <u>Cochrane</u> looked at modeling studies, which are inherently inaccurate, to assess the benefit of societal quarantines in reducing deaths and hospitalizations in COVID-19. In the final analysis, they concluded that quarantines are likely effective, but the nature of the quarantine and how it is implemented will determine whether it is successful in slowing disease spread and curbing death.

In COVID-19 communication and policy, quarantines have been deemed necessary and effective, but rarely do experts address the uncertainly of their implementation and duration. More concerning is that the risk of prolonged quarantines is rarely weighed against their uncertain benefit. **Often experts ascribe the negative consequences of quarantines not to the quarantine but to COVID-19 itself. This is an inaccurate and troubling way to assess risk in health care.**

For instance, we know that in many diseases (we will take the example of high blood pressure), the disease has certain risks, and the treatment has certain risks and benefits. If someone becomes dizzy and faints from a high blood pressure medicine, we don't connect that outcome to the disease, but rather to our treatment of the disease. In that case, we would likely change treatments.

Thus, when describing the detrimental effects of quarantine, we cannot label them as outcomes from COVID-19, but rather from our treatment of COVID-19, which is the quarantine. Only then can we assess the true risks and benefits of our treatments. In the context of quarantines, COVID-19 communication has failed us in this regard.

What data do we have about the adverse effects of quarantines? There is a lot of uncertainty about this. In the school closing and nursing home chapters, we described some of the potential adverse effects of locking up students and vulnerable elders and depriving them of social interaction, exercise, and other activities that in the past were essential to their well-being. Do we have any hard data?

Much of what we know is either speculative or based on self-reported data, and not all of it can be put into a BRCT. However, it is crucial that when experts and others communicate about the impact of prolonged quarantines they describe the uncertainty regarding deleterious effects and don't attribute those effects to COVID-19; they should be honest about the effects being a consequence of our treatment.

In our Springer Nature book about COVID-19 communication, we describe in detail what we know and don't know about the harmful effects of quarantines. But clearly, despite a paucity of data now, it would be irresponsible and inaccurate to attribute all excess deaths that occur this year to COVID-19, since the quarantine itself may well be responsible for deaths and illness that must be distinguished from COVID-19 deaths. At this point, we simply do not know the extent of our treatment's harm.

It is felt that millions worldwide will become impoverished from quarantines. In the United States, hundreds of thousands likely will die from a failure to obtain proper medical care, social isolation, income loss, suicide, and domestic violence, among other causes. Already a dramatic rise in depression and other mental health illnesses can be seen. None of this can be tied directly to COVID-19; it is all a side effect from our treatment, and honest communication must be clear about that.

Out of 1,000 people subjected to quarantine, there is no data to support or dispute that any lives will be saved from COVID-19 infection.

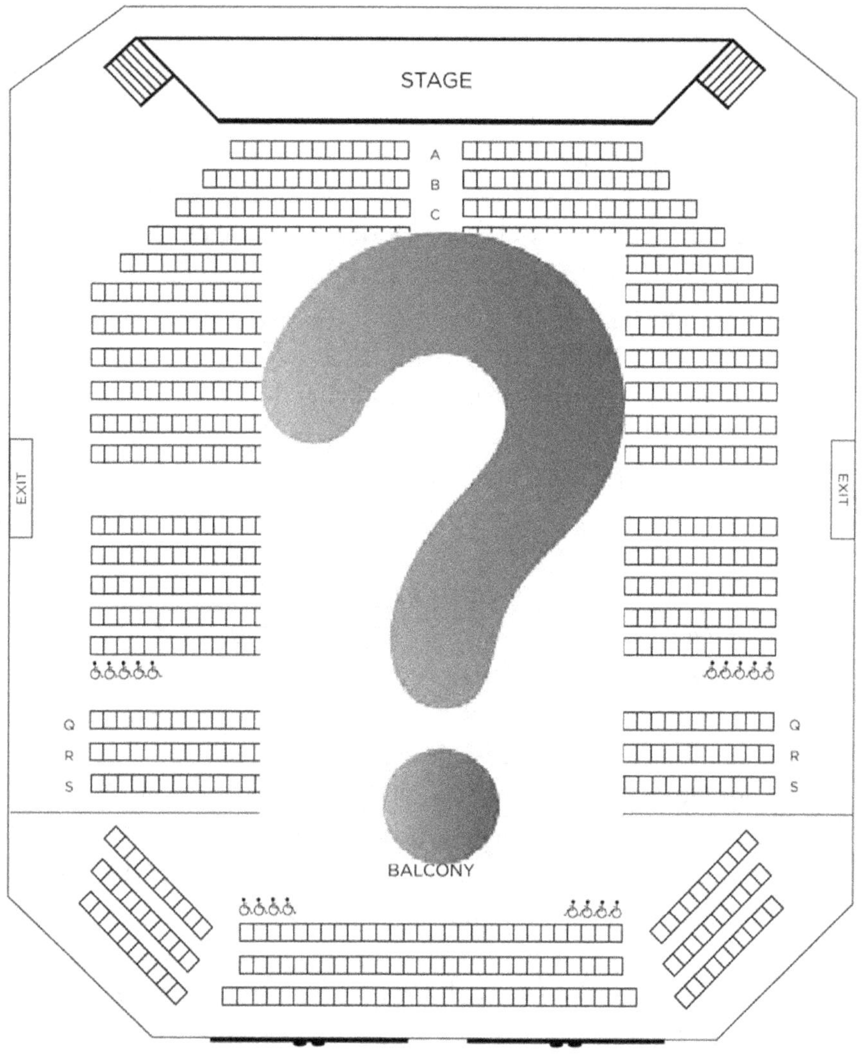

Out of 1,000 people subjected to quarantine, we do not have any data to tell us how many, if any, will suffer from death, physical illness, or mental illness from the quarantine.

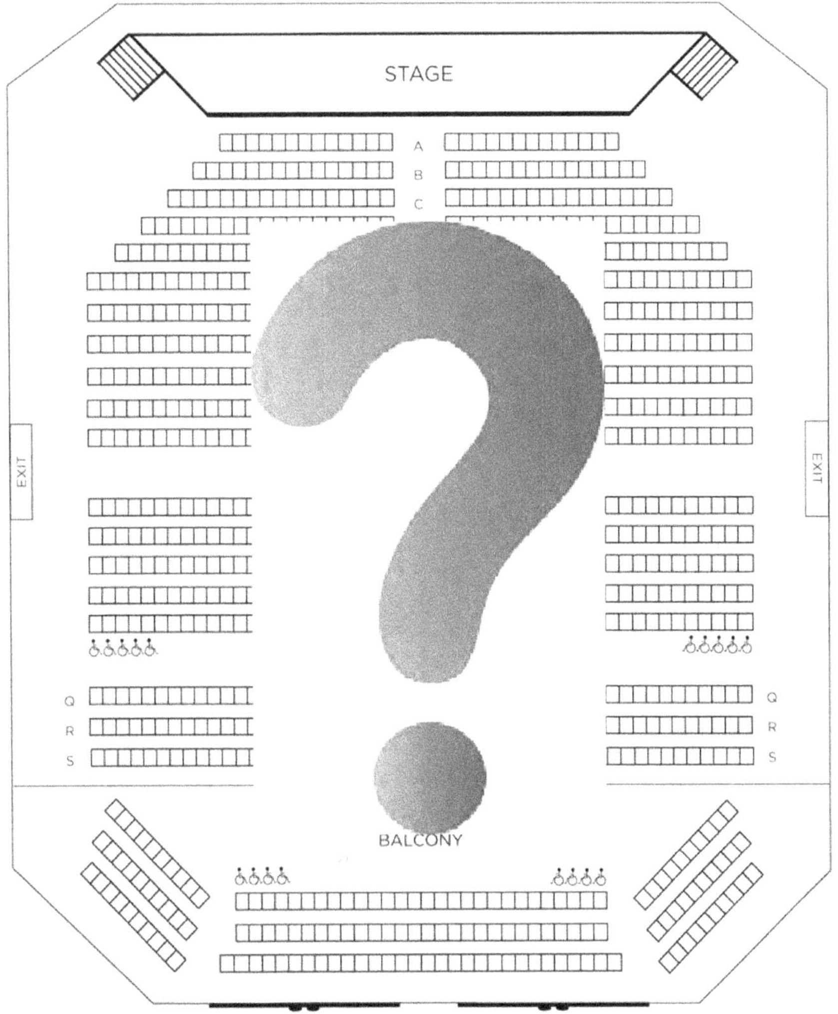

Out of 1,000 people who have lived through the COVID-19 quarantine, 200 report an increase in depressive symptoms compared to the same time last year.

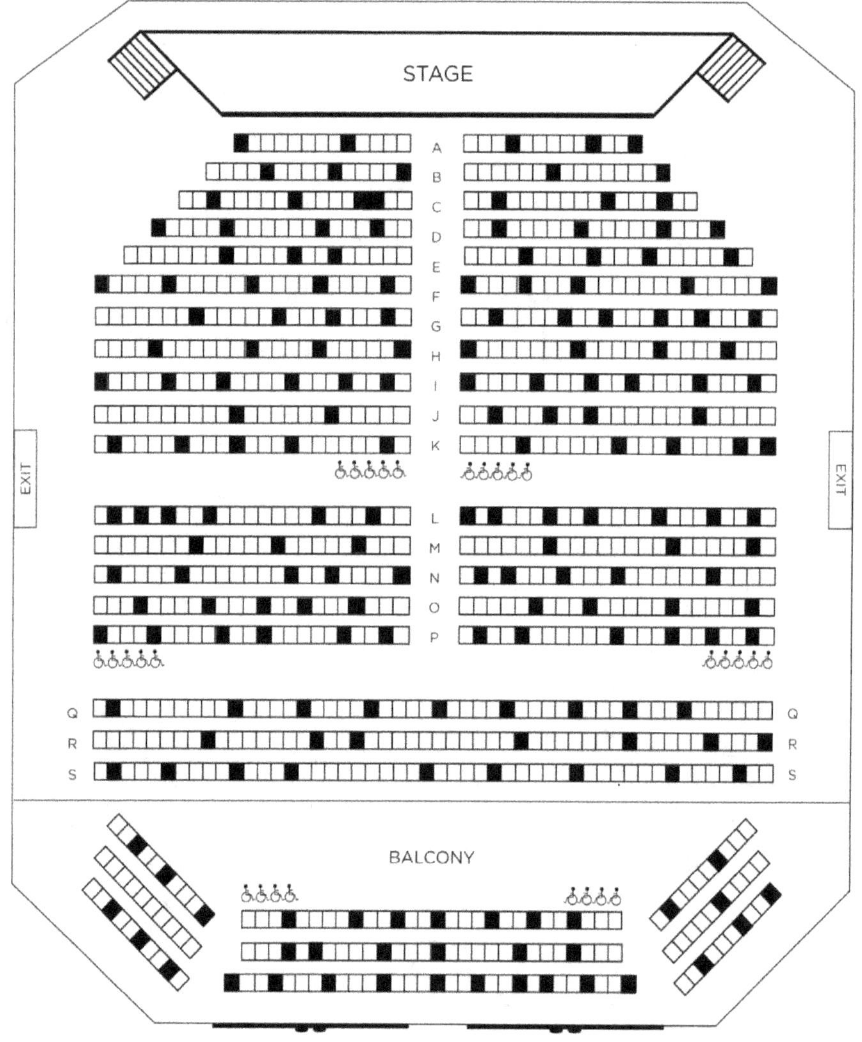

Out of 1,000 people with a history of substance abuse who have lived through the quarantine, 350 report an increase in substance abuse during the quarantine compared to the same time last year.

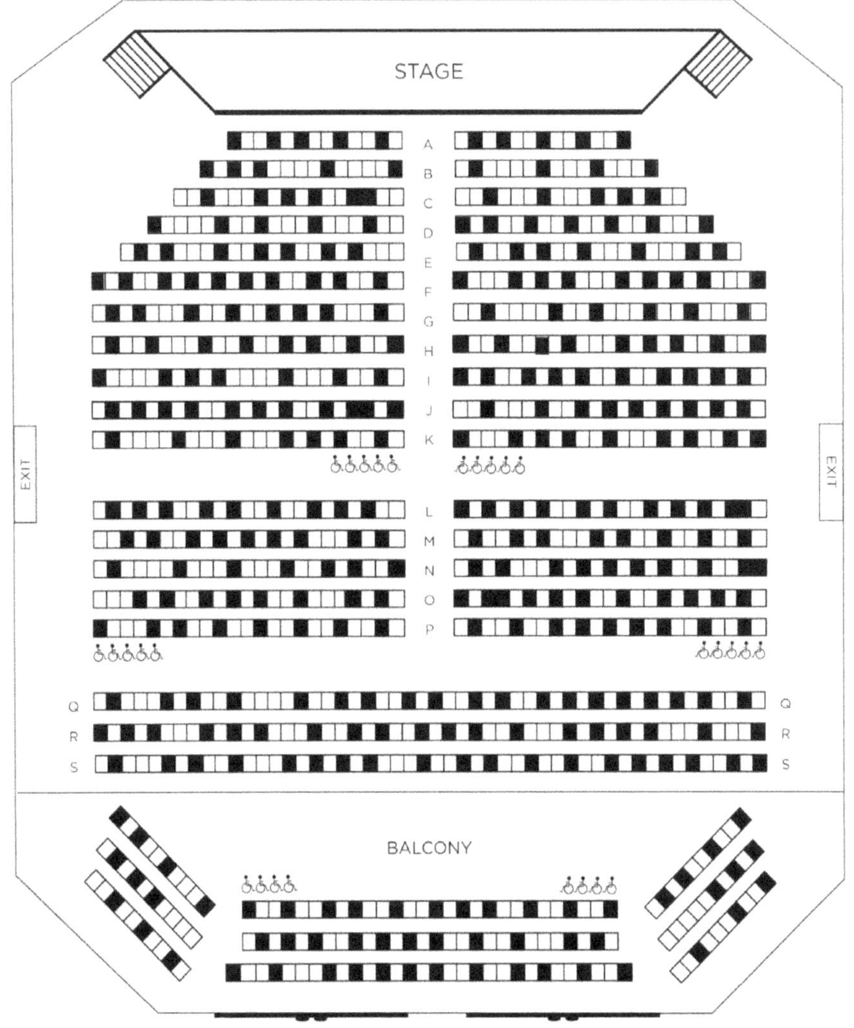

Out of 1,000 people during the quarantine, 530 reported a decline in their mental health compared to the same time last year.

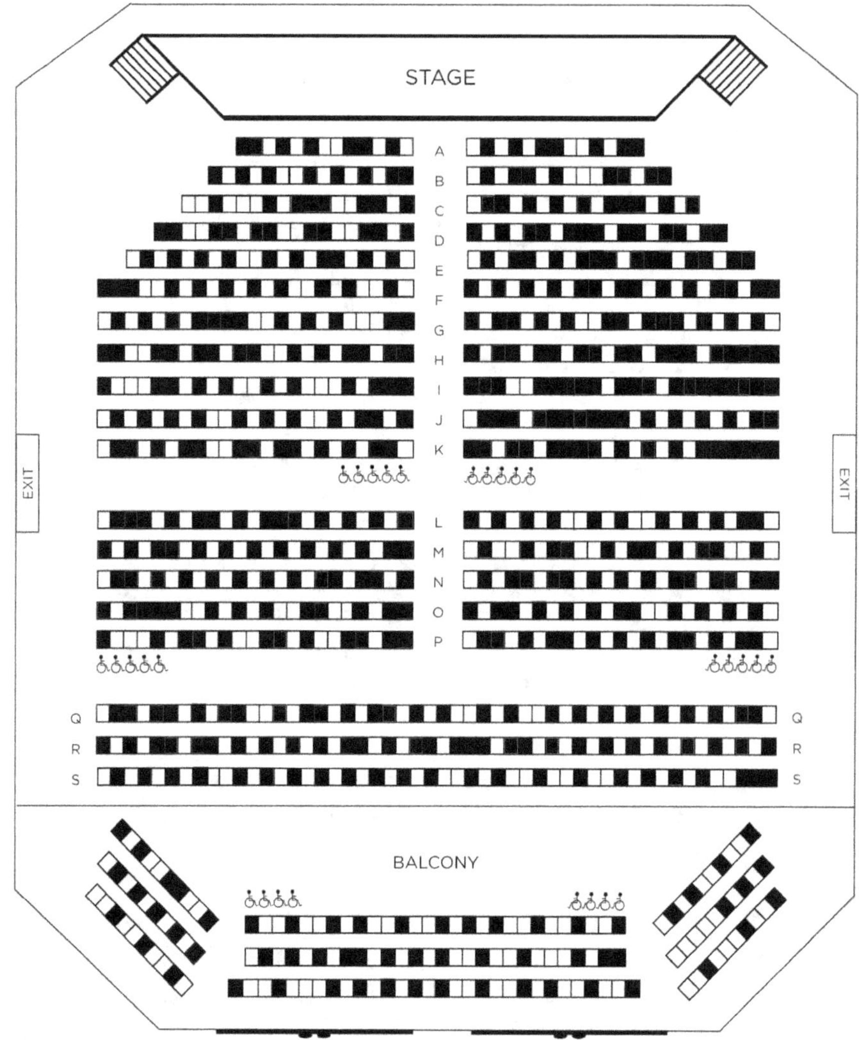

SUMMARY

In COVID-19, societal quarantines and rules to mandate a variety of closures have been a mainstay of policy, many of which have been enforced for over a year. While experts declare unequivocally that these measures are necessary and proven to be effective, we have, in fact, no data from this pandemic or from past viral outbreaks to support that contention, even if it seems that certain restrictions may help curb disease.

The best we can say is that we don't know. Contrarily, few experts have tied the deleterious effects of a prolonged quarantine to the quarantine itself; most blame COVID-19, which is both inaccurate and counterproductive. With any treatment, it is crucial we understand the benefit and risk of the intervention, or else we will be unable to assess its efficacy and harm.

That is also true with the COVID-19 quarantine. How many people has it saved? How many people has it caused to die and be ill? We are currently unsure. We do know that there has been an increase in mental illness and excess deaths during the pandemic. It would be negligent to tie those to COVID-19, which is often inferred from expert communication. Rather, we must assume that at least some of the excess deaths, suffering, and mental illness are from our treatment, and we must make efforts to better delineate the extent of this. Only then can we assess the risks and harms of our treatment. Some points to consider are as follows:

- We are currently uncertain if prolonged quarantines are effective in reducing deaths and hospitalization from COVID-19. We also don't know if more generalized quarantines are useful, or if they should target specific groups and populations. Finally, we are unsure how long a quarantine should be in effect, and whether it can be lifted and reinstated periodically. All of these uncertainties should be conveyed by those communicating about COVID-19 because it is crucial we know what we don't know.
- It has been speculated that prolonged quarantines may cause hundreds of thousands—perhaps millions—of deaths from

starvation, loss of income, failure to get proper medical help due to fear of leaving home, social isolation (especially among elders in long-term care), suicide, domestic violence, and drug/alcohol abuse. All excess deaths that occur during the pandemic must be carefully studied so we can better understand how many were from the disease and how many were from our treatment of the disease. Currently, we don't know how this breaks down, and that uncertainty needs to be better communicated by experts.

* We do know that there has been a dramatic rise in mental illness during the pandemic, and most cases, if not all, have been directly linked to quarantine. Self-reported mental illness and depression—as well as increased suicides, drug abuse, and domestic violence—have been reported and quantified to some extent, but more work must be done. Again, these effects are from our treatment, not from the disease itself, and communication must be clear about that.

* Policy decisions and state-declared mandates based on speculation, and which ignore the potential adverse consequences of our treatment, are the result of poor communication about COVID-19. It is likely that we could have a more effective approach to fight COVID-19 if we are honest and open about our treatments, including their uncertainty and the potential harms.

CHAPTER 6

What we know about other infection outbreaks and why communication about that is important

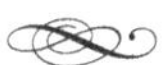

DESPITE WHAT MANY ARE LED to believe by our often sensationalized communication regarding COVID-19, this disease is not the only one we have grappled with in the last hundred years, nor is it necessarily the worst. It is the first one that triggered prolonged societal shutdowns, mandated universal mask use and school closings, and led to various other top-down approaches that we have already discussed. How severe were these other infections, and why did COVID-19 precipitate such a draconian and unheralded response? What can we learn from how the world responded to other similar outbreaks?

Unfortunately, the message both implicit and explicit in COVID-19 communication is, "This is not the flu." And yet, while COVID-19 killed 2.5 million people worldwide in 2020, the 1918 influenza outbreak killed the equivalent of 300 million people at the time, and outbreaks in 1957 and 1968 and even in 2017 killed a similar number of people as COVID-19, many of whom were younger and less frail.

Thus, in severing the current pandemic from Influenza outbreaks to which COVID-19 is similar—both are spread through respiratory carriage and both viruses are of similar size, and thus masks and other preventive measures would be similarly effective/ineffective in both—our COVID-19 experts and the media emphatically dismissed anyone who dared suggest that we could learn from the flu, consistently proclaiming that COVID-19 is unique and more severe. This deprived us of heeding the lessons of the past and putting our current pandemic in a historical perspective, both of which could have helped us to confront COVID-19 more rationally, scientifically, and humanistically.

The 1918 influenza outbreak, which was particularly virulent against the young, killing 10 percent of all young adults/kids and 5 percent of all people on the planet, spread similarly to COVID-19. It disseminated most rapidly in crowded venues, such as military bases and at parades—it struck at the end of the First World War—and could surge through a dense population quickly, killing a large percentage of people it struck. Attempts to curb its spread through quarantines and with mandatory mask use all failed; these have been well studied. Only by stopping large gatherings did the virus kill less rapidly, and only when it finally mutated (it transformed into what today's experts call a variant) did it become inert.

Large influenza outbreaks in 1957 and 1968 hit the world with a similar voracity. In both outbreaks there were no school closings, societal shutdowns, or mandatory mask laws; it was clear by then that masks were not effective against influenza. In 1957, the flu death toll worldwide was similar to what it is with COVID-19, but it was a more lethal virus.

While 3/1,000 people who acquire COVID-19 die, the 1957 flu killed 6.7/1,000 infected people, and it caused serious long-term "long hauler" complications in 30/10,000 people, many of whom were younger. In 1968, the flu death toll worldwide by today's population count would be between 4 and 5 million, almost double the COVID-19 numbers. It was as lethal as the 1957 flu strain but was particularly deadly to younger people and kids, very much unlike COVID-19. Both of these outbreaks fizzled away without intervention. A flu outbreak 3 years ago, in 2017, also was more lethal than COVID-19 to kids and young adults and similarly killed about 2.5 million people worldwide. There were no mandated restrictions or closures in the wake of this virulent strain.

Yes, COVID-19 is not flu, but when experts fail to acknowledge the similarity of disease spread, death rates, and prevention measures with past influenza outbreaks, they are preventing us from realizing that COVID-19 is not unique, and it likely will not be mitigated with our current strategies. This has been yet another failure of communication in the pandemic.

Out of 1,000 people who were infected with COVID-19 across the entire population, 3 of them succumbed to the illness.

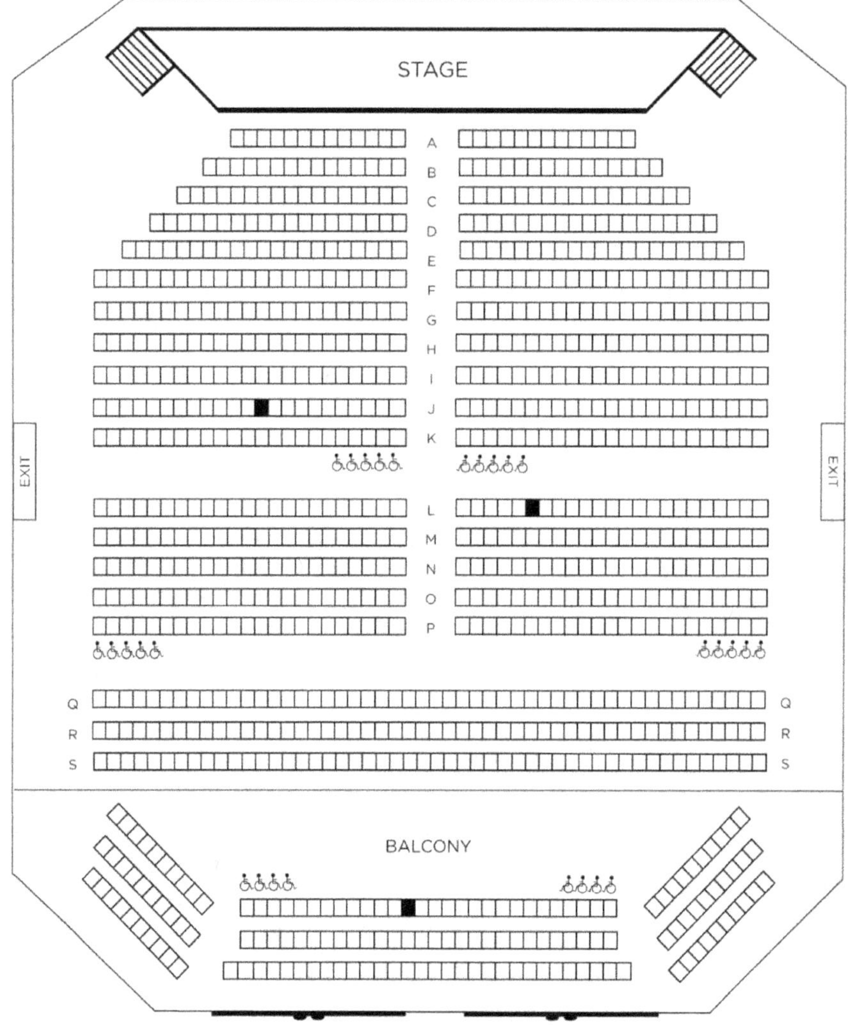

Out of 1,000 people infected with influenza in 1957, 6 of them succumbed to the illness.

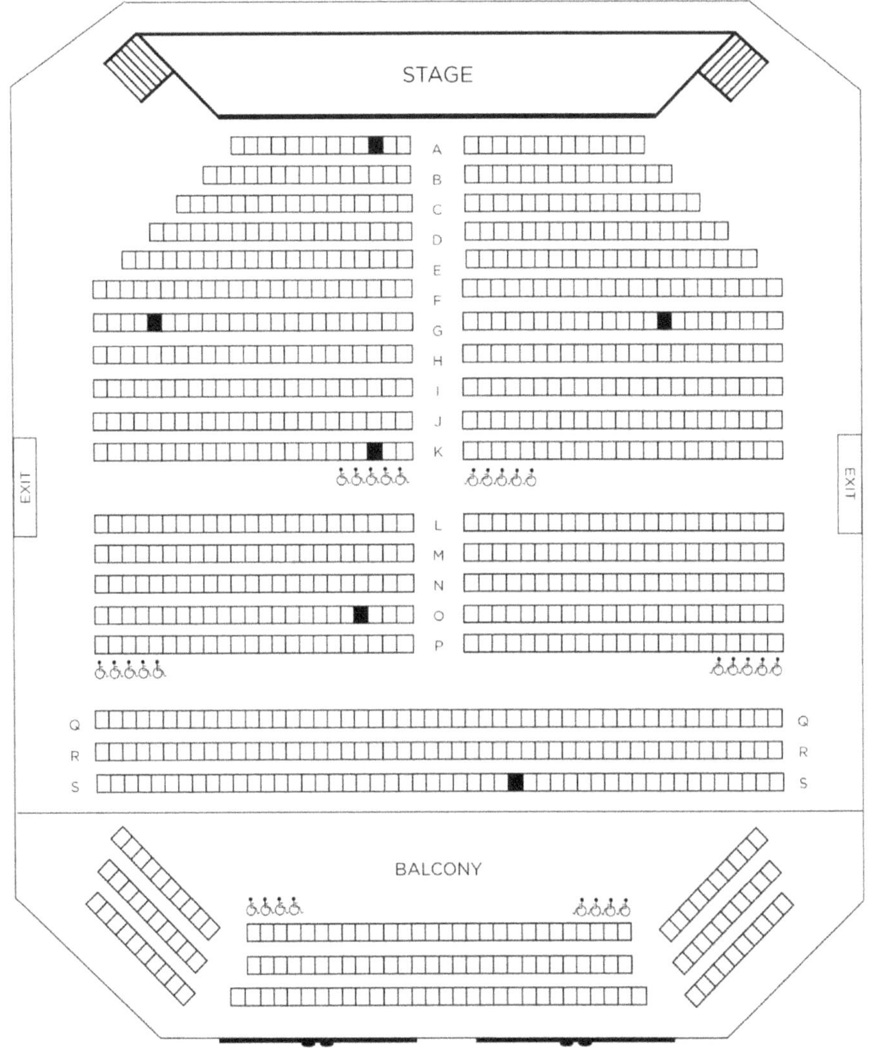

Out of 1,000 people infected by influenza in 1918, 25 succumbed to the illness.

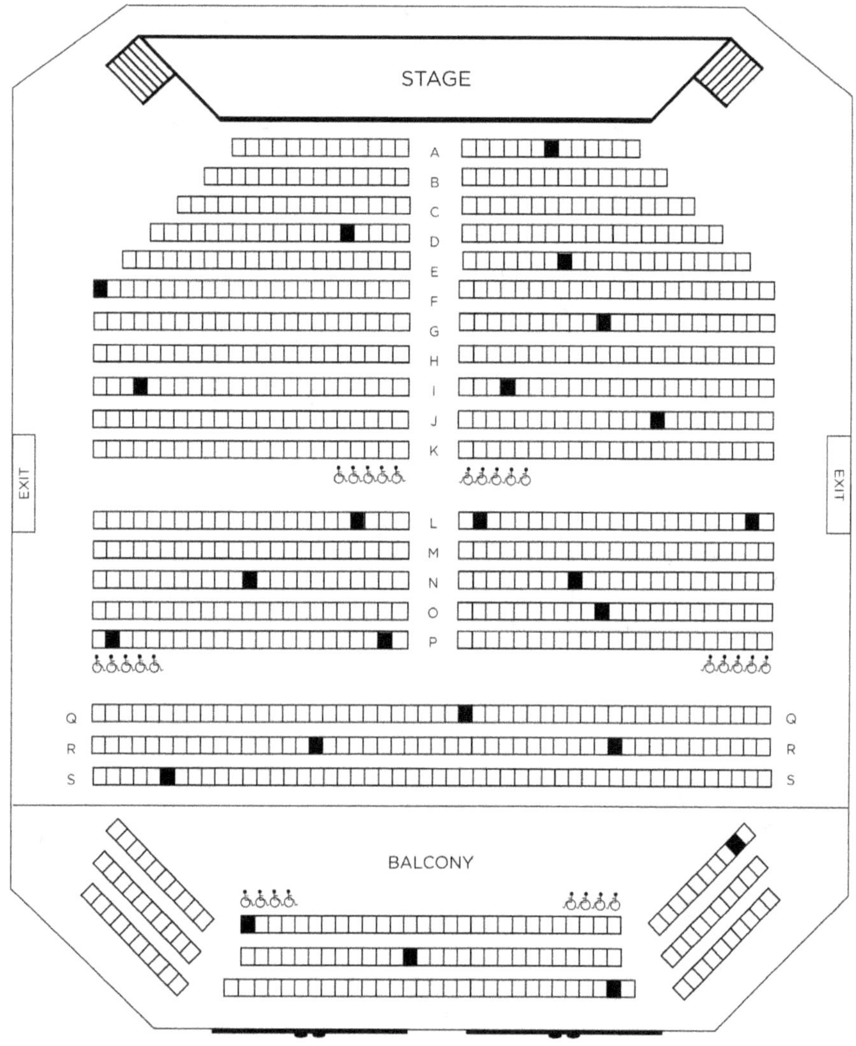

The next three pages depict the death rate of various infections. The first page shows the death rate of COVID-19 (2.5/10,000), the second page the death rate from the 1968 influenza epidemic (12/10,000), and the third page the death toll of the 1918 pandemic (230/10,000). This helps compare COVID-19 to other infectious outbreaks in the past century.

Out of 10,000 people during the COVID-19 pandemic, 2.5 died of the infection.

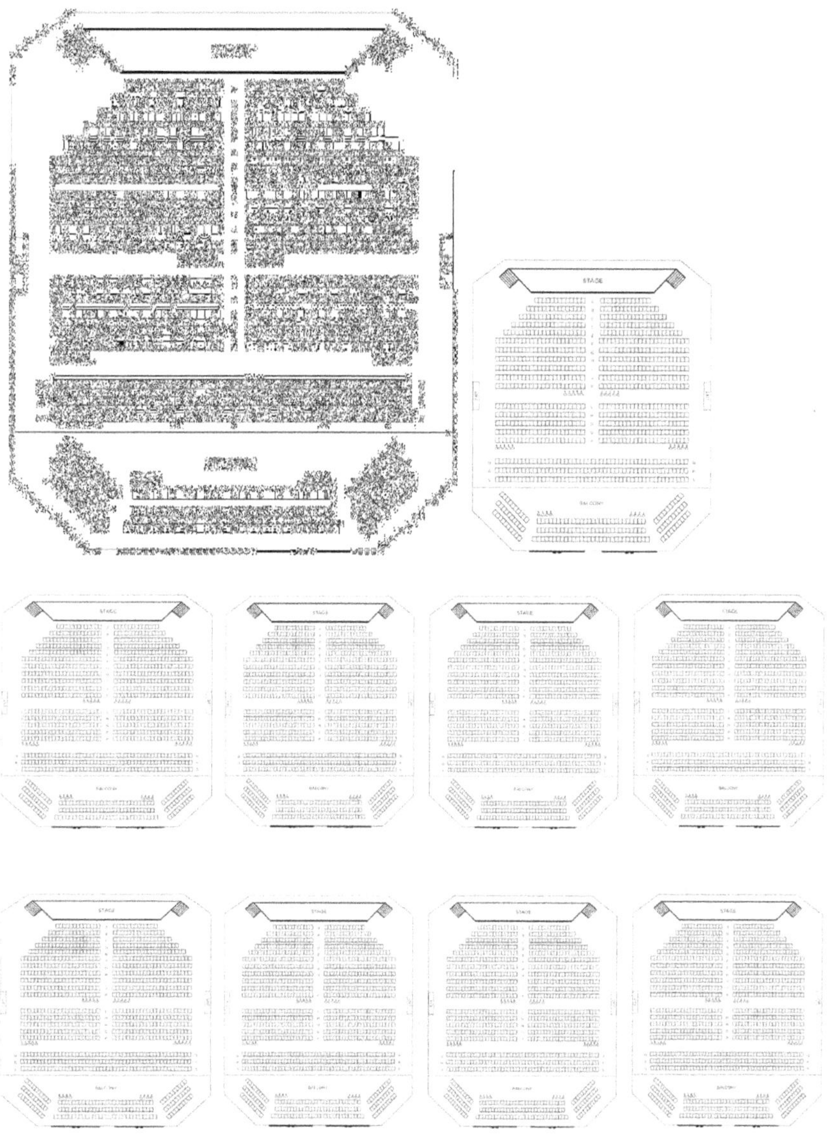

Out of 10,000 people during the 1968 influenza epidemic, 12 died of the infection.

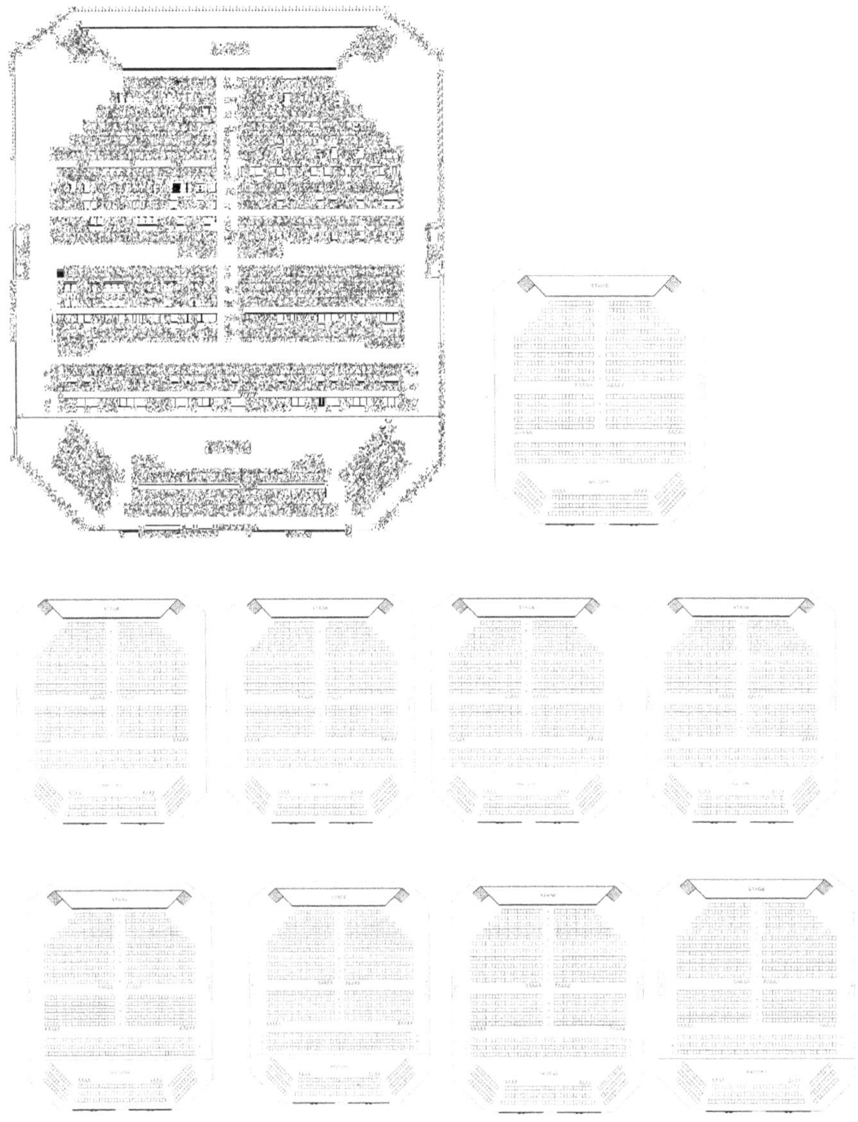

Out of 10,000 people during the 1918 influenza pandemic, 230 died of infection.

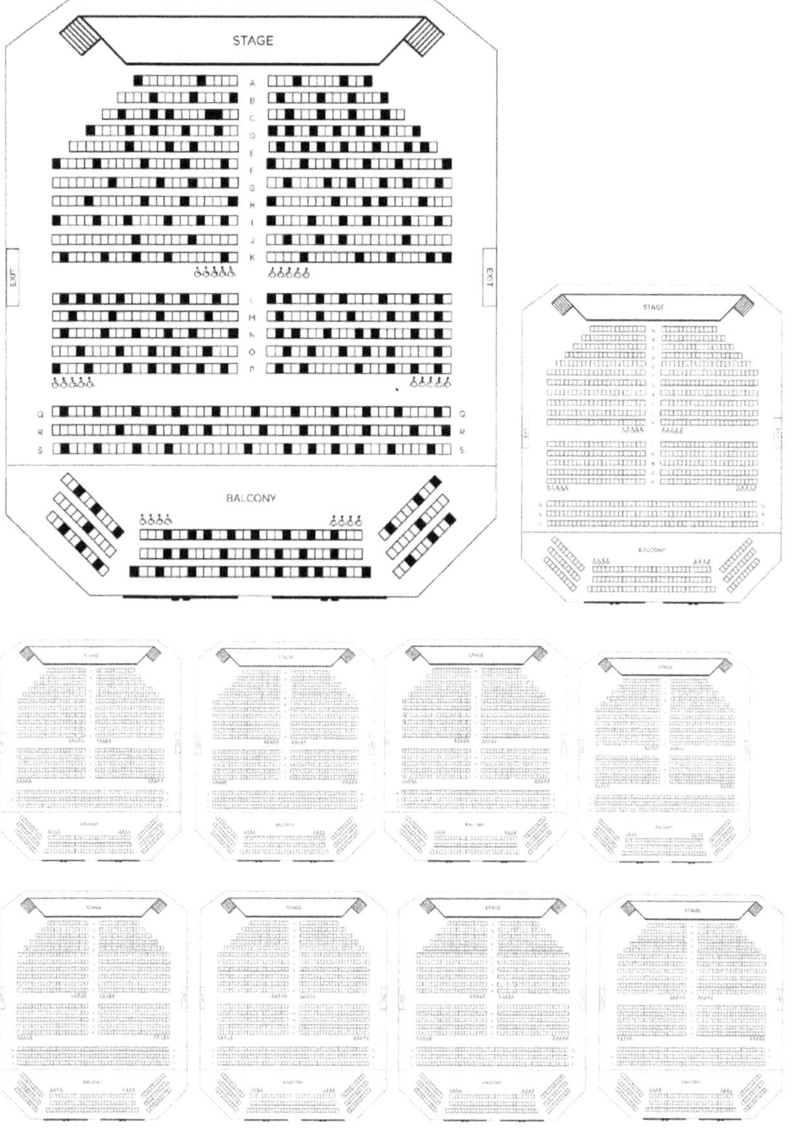

Out of 1,000 people who wore masks during the 1918 influenza epidemic compared to 1,000 people who didn't wear masks, no lives were saved.

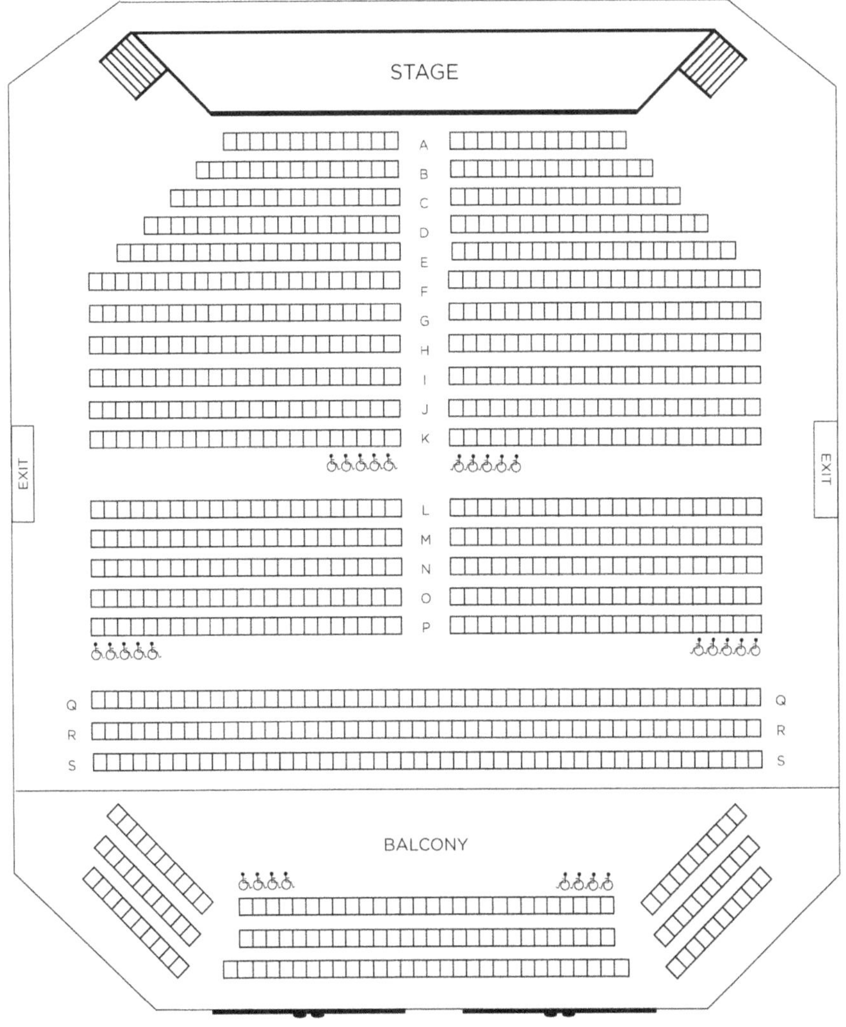

SUMMARY

While it is almost sacrilege to compare COVID-19 to influenza, and while experts and the media refuse to discuss other viral outbreaks and contend that COVID-19 is far worse than anything we have seen in the last 100 years, such communication both obscures the reality of past viral outbreaks and prevents us from learning from them.

Influenza is of a similar size to COVID-19 and spreads in the same manner, and strategies to protect people from the virus and to curb viral spread have similar efficacy in influenza and COVID-19. Thus, we should be honest about the severity, spread, and treatments in past outbreaks. In this chapter we have looked at several flu outbreaks with similar mortality to COVID-19, and one with higher mortality.

The lessons learned from these could have constructively influenced how we reacted to COVID-19 and helped us to put this pandemic in perspective, rather than labeling it as a uniquely lethal viral outbreak that behaves differently than flu. In fact, had we looked to the past, we may well have faced this pandemic more scientifically and sensibly, something that the prevailing COVID-19 communication prevented us from doing. A few salient points are given below:

- The 1918 influenza epidemic was far more deadly than COVID-19, killing a significantly larger number of infected people and a larger percentage of the population. Attempts to curb it by mask use were ineffective; only avoiding large gatherings seemed to slow its spread.
- The flu epidemics of 1957 and 1968 killed a similar number of people worldwide as COVID-19—the 1968 flu was more pernicious, especially to younger people—and was more deadly than COVID-19 for those who were infected. Again, masks and other top-down measures were deemed ineffective.
- A particularly deadly flu outbreak in 2017, just three years ago, killed a similar number of people worldwide as COVID-19 did in 2020, and was far more deadly to young adults and kids. Despite

this, little attention was given to this outbreak, and no attempts were made to mandate mask use, school closures, or societal shutdowns. For some reason, this outbreak, despite its severity and its similarity in spread to COVID-19, never triggered any large-scale media coverage or governmental response.

* By studying these other outbreaks, and learning why we reacted more severely to some and not others, and learning what measures helped to slow the spread and reduce mortality and what measures didn't, we could have approached COVID-19 more rationally.
* **Yes, COVID-19 is not the flu, but it is from the flu that we can learn the most about it.**

CHAPTER 7

Current treatments for COVID-19: what we know and what we don't

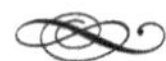

DURING THE PANDEMIC, TREATMENT STRATEGIES have evolved that have, to some extent, reduced the chance of dying of COVID-19. Early on, it was unclear how to treat it. Hospitalization was not effective, and intubation was a death sentence much of the time. Even today, many COVID-19 patients who are considered to have moderate to severe disease—mostly due to drops in their oxygen levels—are hospitalized without much evidence that the hospital is helpful or necessary in many cases. In the hospital, and even out of the hospital, novel treatments are now being used to reduce death and to lower the need for ventilators. How effective are they?

Early in the crisis, much hype circulated about several medicines like hydroxychloroquine and certain vitamin cocktails. These treatments were largely dismissed by experts, and subsequent studies showed them to be ineffective, although the studies were done in hospital patients who had more advanced disease.

As the mechanism of death in COVID-19 became clearer—which, had we studied in past flu outbreaks, we could have ascertained much earlier in the pandemic—other treatments evolved, mostly to address the hyper-inflammatory state induced by COVID-19 (the use of steroid) and the tendency to get blood clots (the use of anticoagulants). While there is much anecdotal evidence regarding the efficacy of these methods, especially in nonhospitalized long-term care patients who are ill, they have not been formally studied in the outpatient arena.

The use of the steroid dexamethasone has been looked at in severe disease among hospitalized patients. It has been shown to reduce deaths in a <u>large clinical trial</u> of people in the hospital with severe disease, most of whom were under 70 years of age. Overall, in 28 days, the use of dexamethasone reduced death by 28/1,000 from COVID-19 between those who took it and those who didn't.

Whether the same results could be achieved by using variable doses in people outside the hospital with more mild illnesses is uncertain. Similarly, basic anticoagulation drugs given before blood clots develop among very ill COVID-19 patients in the hospital resulted in 40/1,000 reduced deaths in <u>one trial</u>, although no trials have reviewed the efficacy of giving these drugs to less ill people in an outpatient setting. Still, in this trial, given that 400/1,000 people who died of COVID-19 had some form of blood clot, it would seem sensible to treat high-risk COVID-19 patients with anticoagulants, even in outpatient settings.

Studies of antiviral intravenous treatments for COVID-19, such as <u>Remdesivir</u>, have shown variable results, typically demonstrating some decrease in disease severity, but no statistically significant reduction in death. There is no benefit of oral antivirals in influenza or COVID-19, although they have not been well studied in the latter.

Monoclonal antibodies, another intravenous treatment that can be given as an outpatient, have also had variable results. Two early studies showed no benefit of these medicines, while a <u>later study</u> that looked at a combination of bamlanivimab and etesevimib showed that, among those people given treatment early in the course of their disease, 20/1,000 fewer people died in the treatment group. There were also fewer hospitalizations by 50/1,000. <u>Other studies</u> have not shown a reduction in death, and such therapy is not without side effects and comes at a high price tag compared to the use of steroids and anticoagulants. It is important to know that these drugs were not compared to steroids, and the studies were not conducted on anyone using steroids.

There are some effective treatments for COVID-19 and others less effective; as to who most benefits, which combinations are most efficacious, and in which venue they should be used—that is currently uncertain.

Out of 1,000 hospitalized patients with severe COVID-19 infection and who were given steroids (dexamethasone) compared to 1,000 who did not receive this, 28 fewer people died.

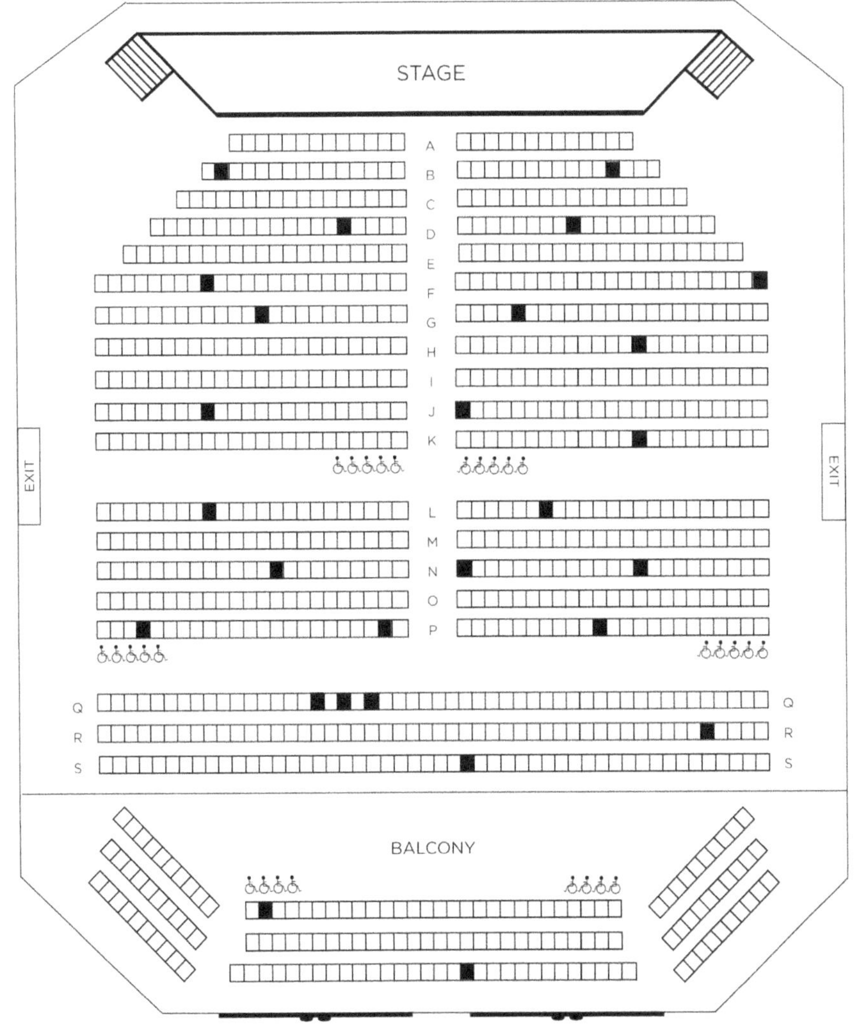

Out of 1,000 hospitalized patients with severe COVID-19 infection and who were given anticoagulation drugs (blood thinners) compared to 1,000 who did not receive this, 40 fewer people died.

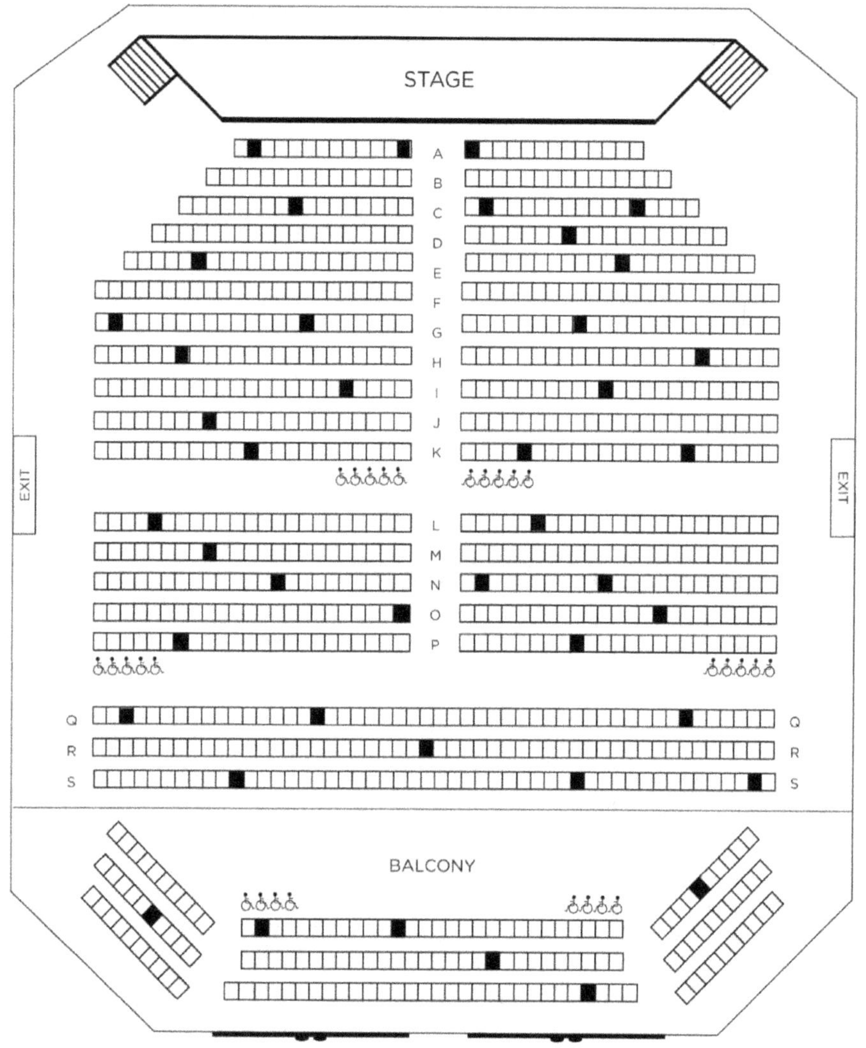

Out of 1,000 people with COVID-19 who died, 400 of them were found to have blood clots which may or may not have contributed to the death, explaining why anticoagulants may be effective in all stages of the disease.

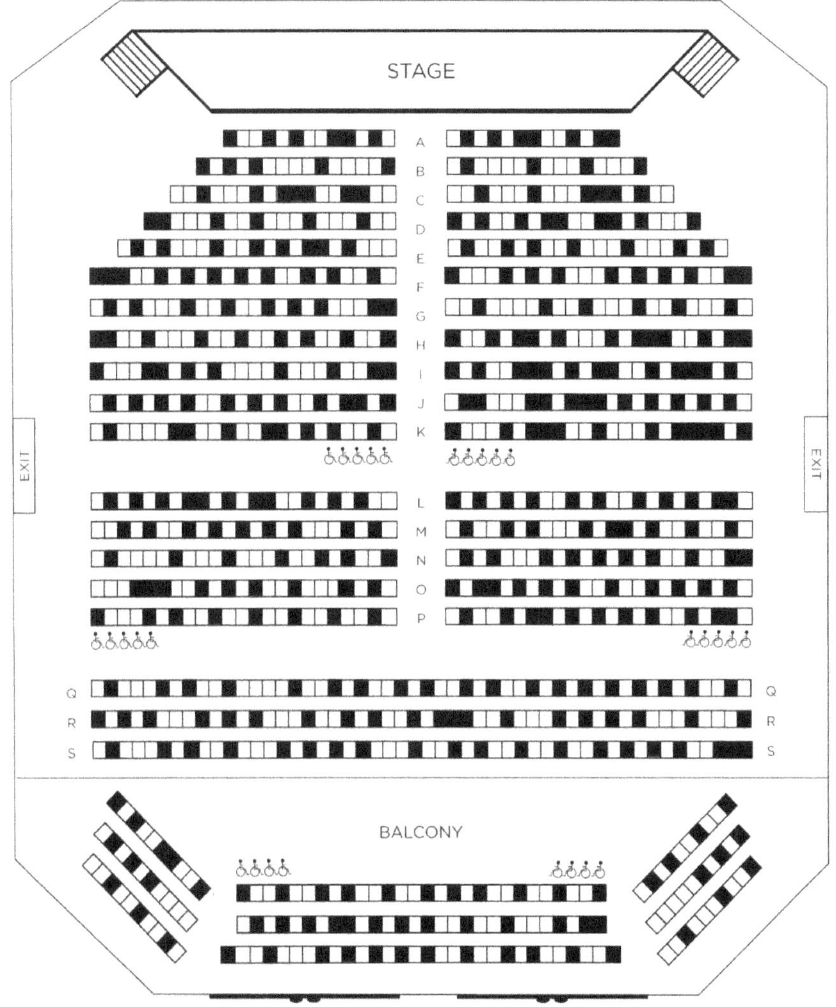

Out of 1,000 patients with COVID-19 infection in the hospital who received intravenous antiviral treatments such as Remdesivir compared to 1,000 not treated, no lives were saved.

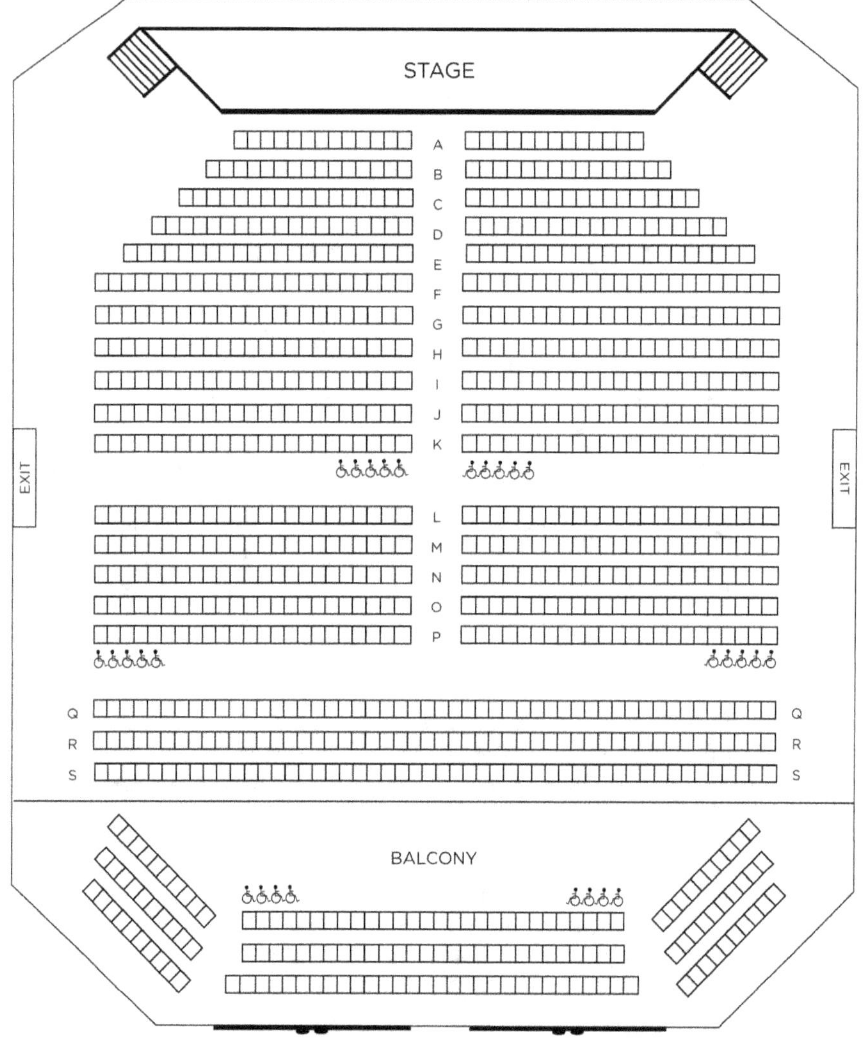

Out of 1,000 patients with COVID-19 infection who received monoclonal antibodies compared to 1,000 who did not, most showed no lives saved, while one study of a combination drug showed 20 lives saved.

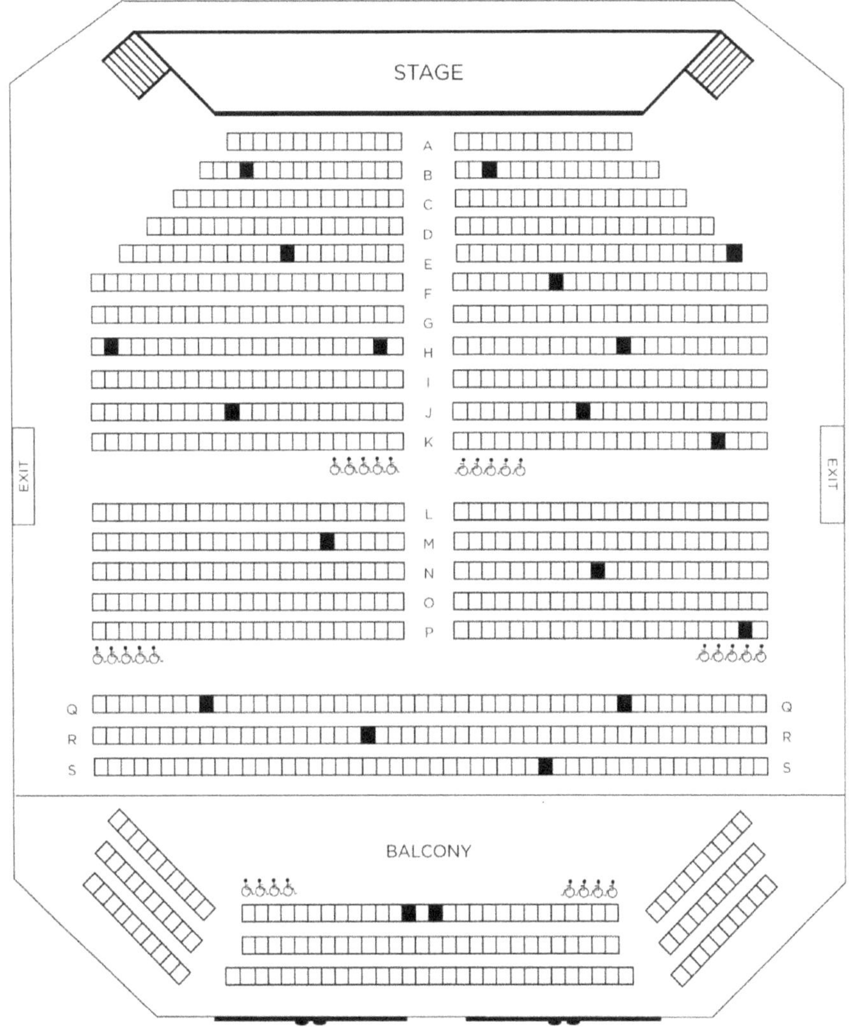

Out of 1,000 people with mild or moderate COVID-19 infection who are not hospitalized, we are not sure if there is any benefit from steroids or anticoagulation; few studies have been done.

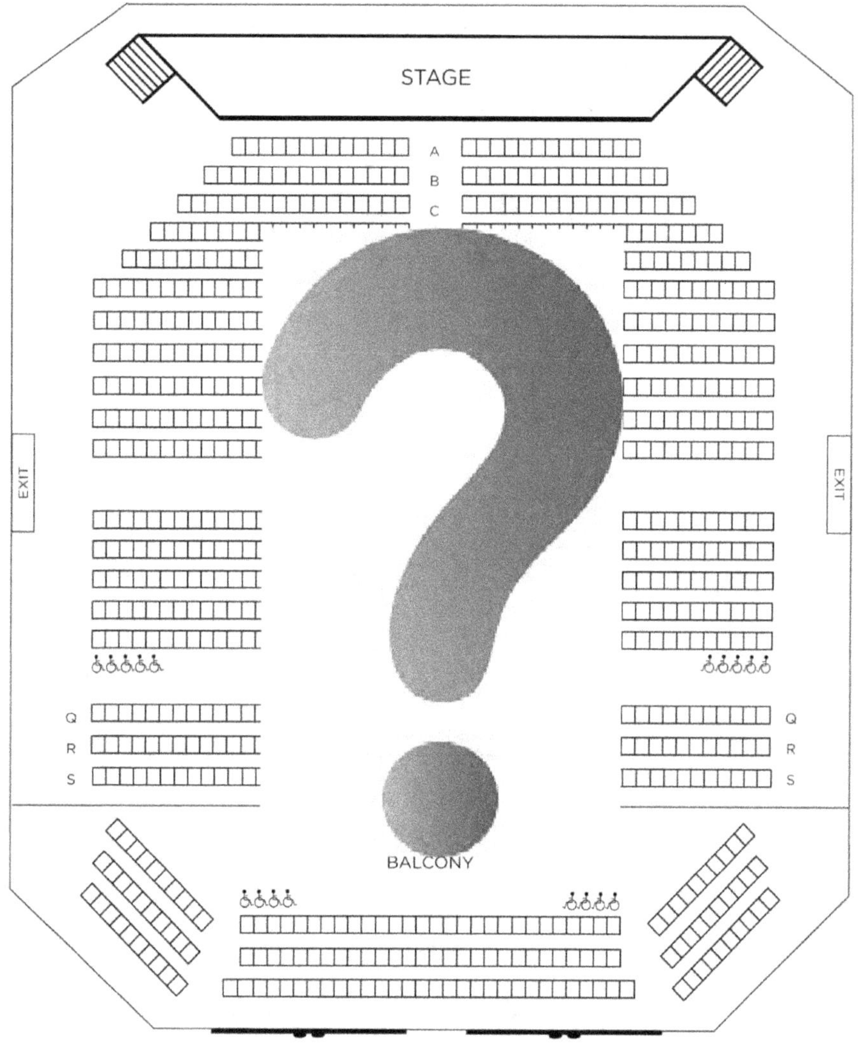

Out of 1,000 people with COVID-19 infection who were hospitalized compared to 1,000 who were not, we do not know if any lives were saved.

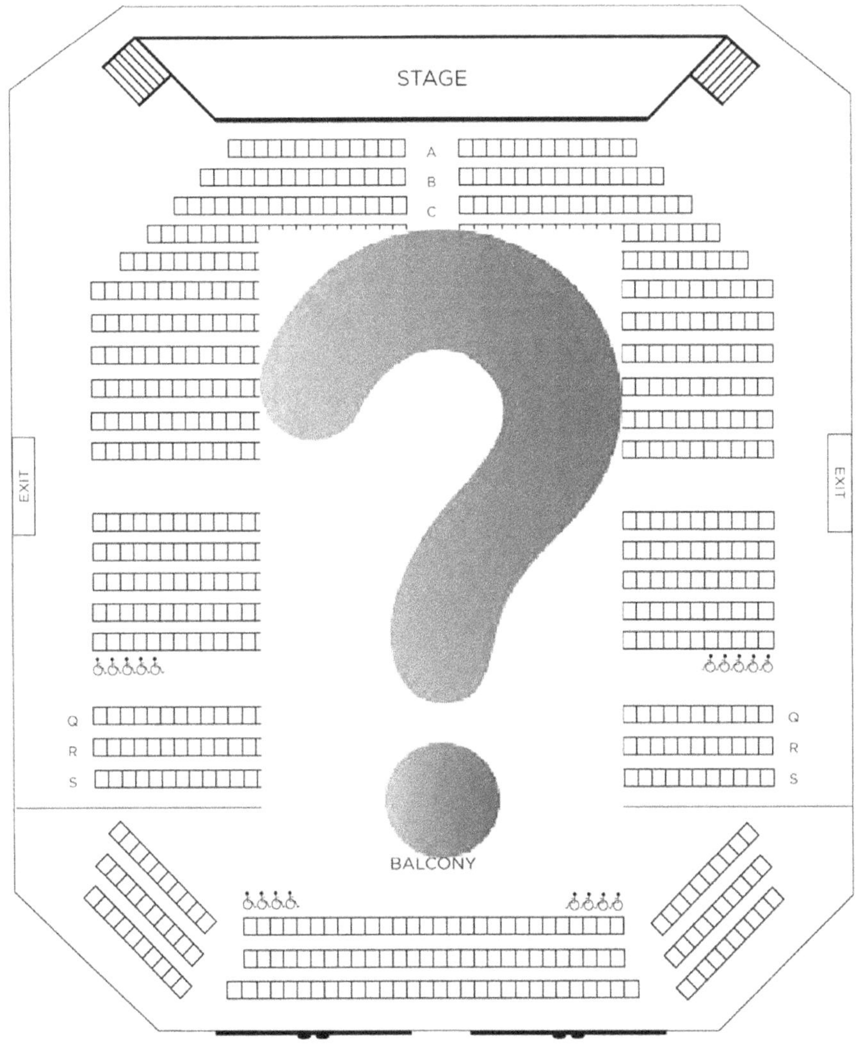

Summary

As the COVID-19 pandemic has progressed, many drug treatments have been studied, and many have not. We know that, similar to other deadly respiratory viral infections, the mechanism of death in COVID-19 is related to the body's hyper-inflammatory response and the tendency to get blood clots, many of which are lethal.

Thus, reducing inflammation and giving medicines to prevent blood clots would seem to be the best approach to take. Studies have shown that the use of steroids and anticoagulants in hospitalized COVID-19 patients with severe disease are effective in reducing deaths, but few similar studies have been conducted in outpatient settings and among less ill high-risk patients.

The use of monoclonal antibodies seems to have variable success, while antiviral treatments do not reduce death; both of these treatment modalities are far more expensive than outpatient steroids and anticoagulants. While many people with moderate to severe COVID-19 are hospitalized, there is no evidence that hospitalization improves the outcome, and it can lead to worse outcomes potentially due to hospital-induced infections and errors/overtreatment. A few salient points are given below:

- Given that the mechanism of death in COVID-19 is related to a hyper-inflammatory state and increased risk of blood clots, the use of steroids and anticoagulants makes clinical sense. One trial showed that 400/1,000 people who died of COVID-19 had blood clots.
- Both steroids and anticoagulants do reduce death in ill hospitalized patients.
- There have been no trials of steroid use and oral anticoagulants in COVID-19 among nonhospitalized patients who are at high risk, mostly those who are elderly and in long-term care. This would seem to be the most important venue of their use.

- There is no evidence that hospitalizing patients at high risk or with moderate disease has any benefit or does it actually increase risk.
- Antivirals do not reduce mortality and can only be given in the hospital.
- Monoclonal antibodies may reduce death when given early in the course of disease; some studies show benefits, some do not.
- It is unclear if monoclonal antibodies are superior to steroids and anticoagulants, or if they can be used in conjunction with those other modalities of treatment, since no study has compared or combined these treatments.
- Monoclonal antibody use renders subsequent vaccination ineffective for three months, and its side effects, especially for the elderly, have not been well defined.
- All treatments must be patient-specific, and often there are no trials that define what is appropriate for the particular patient who is being treated.
- Most drug trials have been conducted in the hospital and do not involve the frail elderly who reside in long-term care; given that these are the most vulnerable people to the effects of COVID-19, the failure to focus on them in studies is a glaring oversight.

CHAPTER 8

The risks and benefits of COVID-19 vaccinations

RECENTLY, THE MOST SALIENT DEVELOPMENT in COVID-19 treatment was related to the availability of vaccination. Now that the vaccine has been introduced and has been disseminated to the most vulnerable people, health care workers, and then more generally, the rates of COVID-19 illness and death have diminished appreciably. There is still a large sector of the community that is skeptical about vaccination and does not fully understand both the mechanism and ramifications of being immunized. In addition, there are several types of vaccines, and the efficacy and risks of each are difficult to fully grasp.

Many experts in COVID-19 believe that the primary goal of generalized immunization is to establish herd immunity. Herd immunity occurs when approximately 80 percent of people are immune to a virus, either by contracting the virus and developing antibodies or by being vaccinated. Currently, CDC estimates that we are close to that threshold, especially since approximately 60 percent of Americans have had COVID-19.

However, herd immunity is not itself a requisite goal of vaccination. We don't attempt to achieve herd immunity in many other common deadly viruses, including influenza, because our goal is narrow: to immunize those most vulnerable and to contain outbreaks when they do occur. Thus, to policymakers and to individuals, the prime objective of vaccination is to reduce the incidence of serious disease and death from COVID-19, while causing the fewest number of side effects from the vaccine.

As with many COVID-19 issues, communication about COVID-19 vaccination has been confusing and often misleading. Most people do not understand the difference between vaccines, what short- and long-term side effects are of vaccination, how effective the vaccines are, how long immunity lasts, whether someone who has had COVID-19 needs to be immunized, and whether the vaccines are worth being given that some experts still demand strict compliance to mask use and social distancing even after vaccination.

Some experts toss out numbers, such as the vaccine being 95 percent effective; while other experts claim that vaccines are not effective against variants and thus being vaccinated does not necessarily protect someone. A recent article in *Science* discusses the statistical confusion that is often the result of pharmaceutical companies and public health agencies trying to amplify the benefits of vaccination, but serving only to confuse people about its risks and benefits.

In fact, suggests author Adam Rogers, "By not being clear about the different flavors of risk and benefit for different vaccines and different people, public health experts have let doubt and dodgy personal interpretations flourish." This is especially true because, as we have shown in this book, the chance of dying from COVID-19 is often very small, especially in younger and healthier people.

Thus, if a vaccine cuts the risk of death down by even as much as 50 percent, that reduction is tiny in actual terms for someone, let's say a student, whose risk of death is only 2 out of 100,000. By not being upfront about who most benefits from vaccination, based mostly on their risk of dying from COVID-19 in the first place, communication about vaccines has sowed enough doubt to promote a culture of vaccine hesitancy.

Some experts also claim that vaccination does not mean that you can take off your mask or hug your parents; society has not opened due to vaccination, and even in long-term care facilities—where vaccination rates are very high and where the quarantine has proven to be lethal and deleterious—vaccination has not persuaded many health departments to open these places up. This, too, has promoted the belief that vaccines can't be very effective, since they don't even protect those people who are vaccinated.

In fact, the benefits and risks of vaccines can be made clear through a BRCT. Moderna, Pfizer, and Johnson & Johnson have all made vaccines and conducted studies on them. The studies only looked at selected subjects—for instance, no pregnant woman, people with autoimmune diseases, or those with prior COVID-19 infections, and few people over the age of 80—but did compile results that can be placed in a BRCT, as we demonstrate on the following pages.

When a person knows his or her own risk of dying of COVID-19 and also assesses his or her risk of spreading disease to others (such as if they work in public service jobs or spend time with vulnerable, unvaccinated people), then the person can juxtapose those risks against the risks and benefits of the vaccine.

Since, as our BRCTs show, the vaccine is very protective to the individual receiving it in preventing serious COVID-19 infection or death, a vaccinated person need not worry about whether herd immunity is achieved or if he/she comes into contact with someone not vaccinated or who has COVID-19. The vaccinated person is protected. Thus, the decision to get a vaccine must be made by individuals after assessing their own risk and benefit, and our BRCTs can help in that decision. The study that preceded the distribution of the Moderna vaccine compared findings from two groups:

* 15,000 people in a placebo group; and
* 15,000 people in an mRNA group (had the Moderna vaccine)

Results of this were as follows:

1. 11 people in the mRNA group have been infected with COVID-19. 185 people in the placebo have been infected with COVID-19 (see graphic below).

2. Severe Cases:

0 cases in the mRNA group.

30 cases in the placebo group (see graphic below).

In a stadium of 15,000 people, 11 who were vaccinated developed COVID-19 infection (first stadium) compared to 185 who were not vaccinated (second stadium).

Out of 15,000 people in the vaccination arm, 11 developed COVID-19 infection

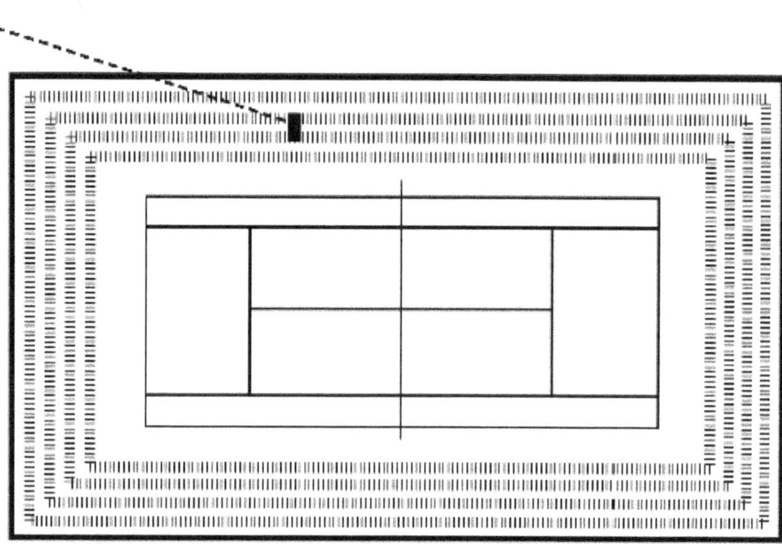

Out of 15,000 people in the placebo arm, 185 developed COVID-19 infection.

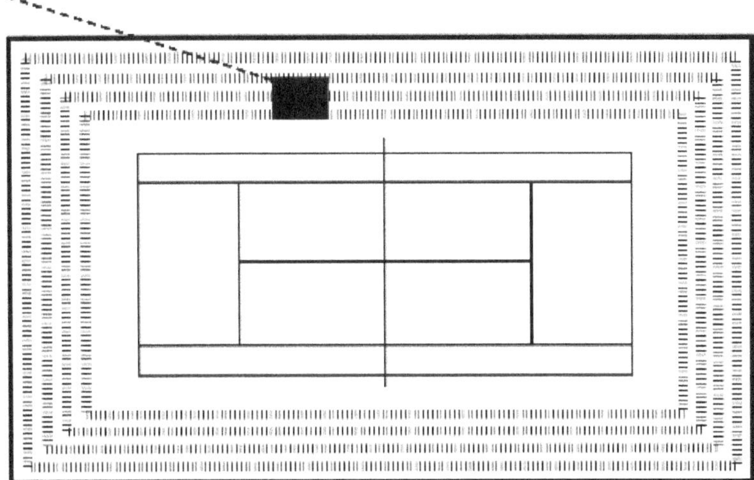

Out of 15,000 people who were vaccinated, none developed severe COVID-19 infection.

0

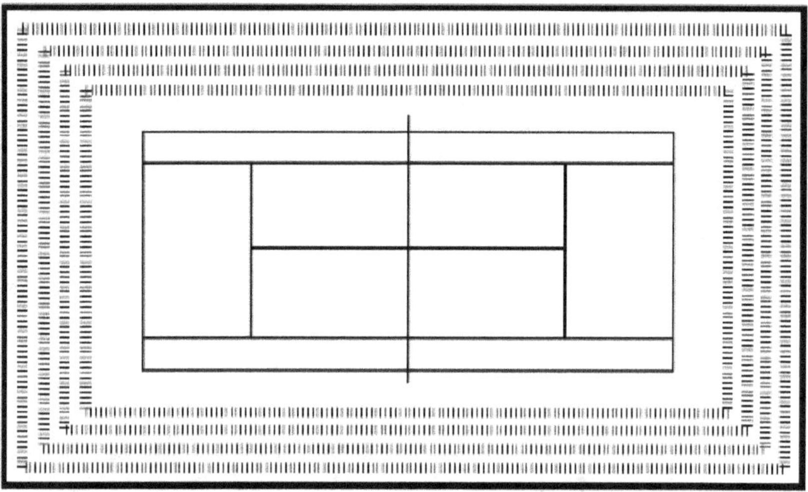

Out of 15,000 people who were not vaccinated, 30 developed severe COVID-19 infection.

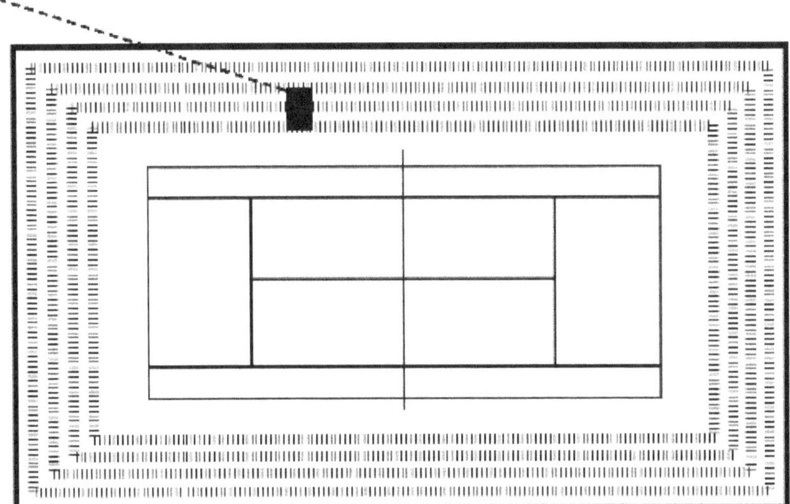

Out of 15,000 people who received the Moderna vaccine, there were no serious side effects.

0

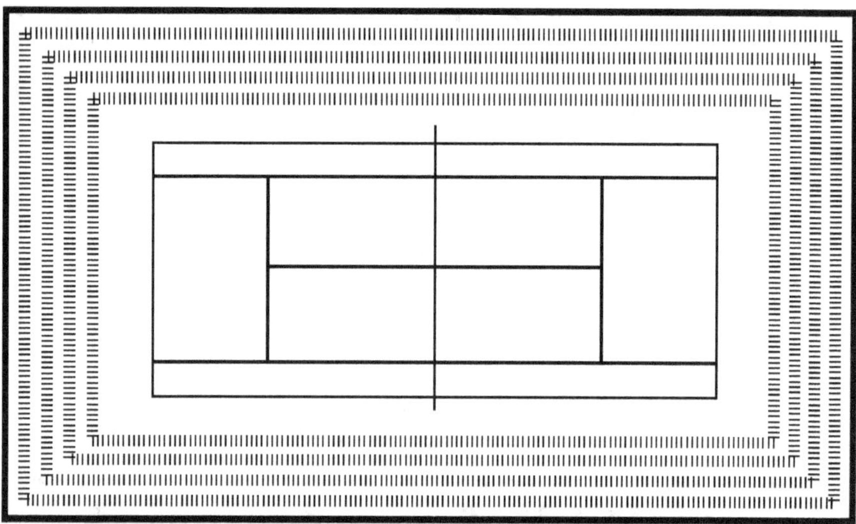

Out of ten 100,000-seat stadiums who received the Johnson & Johnson vaccine, one developed a blood clot, which is the same number who would be hit by lightning in a year.

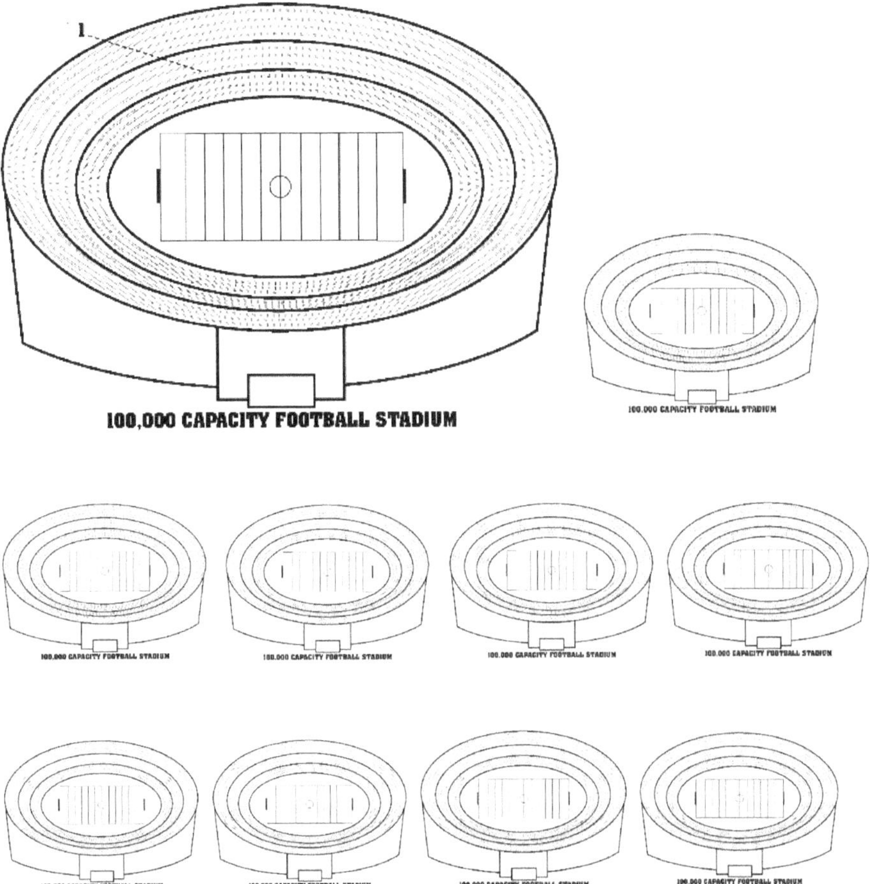

Out of a stadium of 1,000 people who took any of the currently available COVID-19 vaccinations, we have no data as to any long-term side effects.

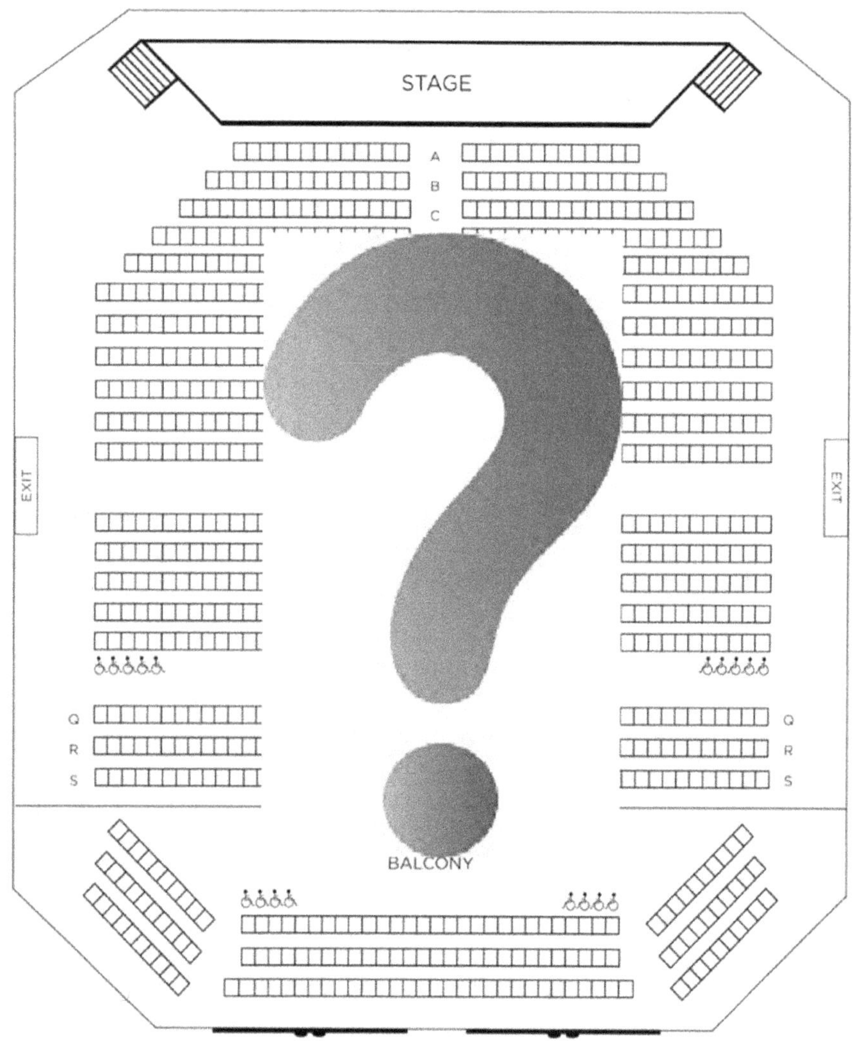

In the Moderna study, there was no difference in severe side effects of the vaccine between the vaccinated and unvaccinated group, meaning no seats were filled in the theater.

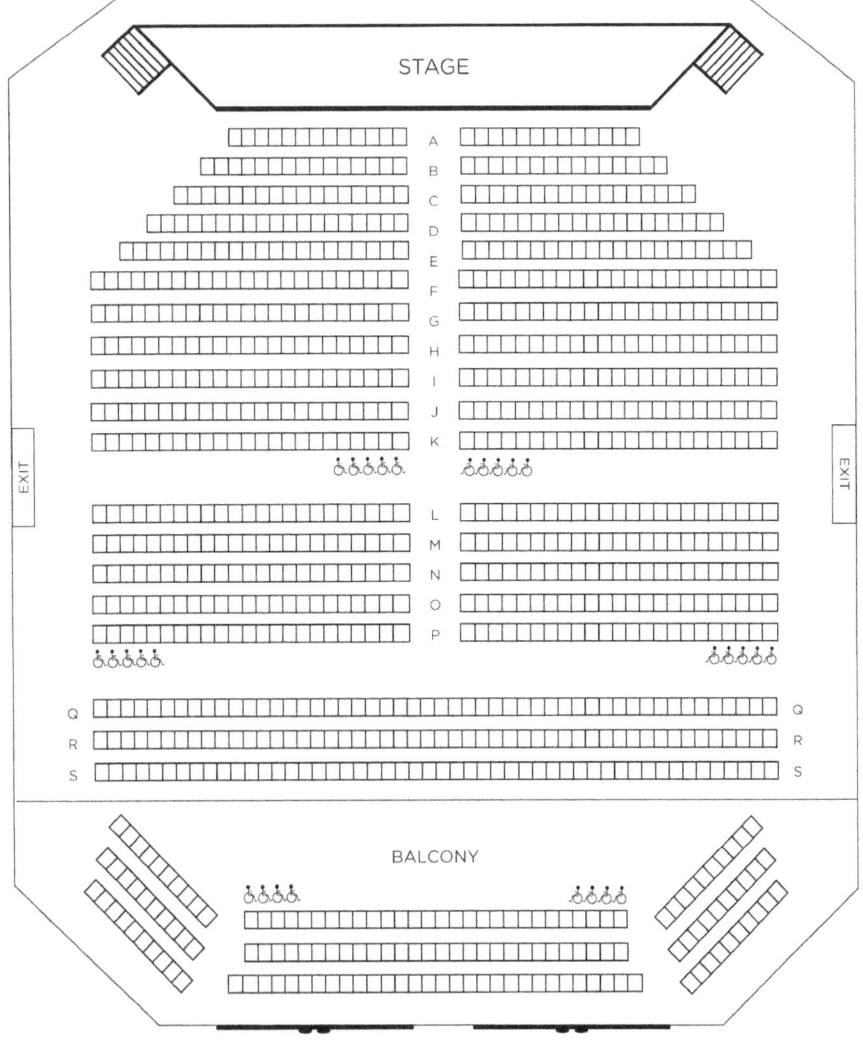

SUMMARY

The decision to get vaccinated must be made by individuals and groups based on their own preferences, their assessment of risk/benefit, and their propensity to spread disease to others. For instance, people who work in restaurants or as teachers may get vaccinated to help them to prevent spreading disease to others, while others will determine whether to get vaccinated based on their own risk of COVID-19.

Thus, there are two parts of any vaccination decision: What is your own risk of disease, and what is your risk of spreading disease to others? We do know what the basic risks and benefits are of vaccination in the short term, as shown on our BRCTs, although long-term risk is impossible to assess given the short duration of vaccine use. The following are salient points:

- The Moderna vaccine has been well studied, and it is felt that Pfizer's vaccine has similar efficacy. The Johnson & Johnson vaccine has a different mechanism of action and may be somewhat less effective, although the actual numbers are difficult to determine.

- With the Johnson and Johnson vaccine, approximately one in a million vaccinated people developed a serious blood clot, which approximates the chance of being hit by lightning this year. It is unclear what the incidence of blood clot is in people not vaccinated, but we do know that COVID-19 itself causes blood clots, so we are unsure if unvaccinated people who get COVID-19 may be at the same or higher risk of clots than vaccinated people.

- Given the short duration of studies and the novel nature of these vaccinations, we are unable to determine long-term side effects or complications. This is represented by a ? on our theater.

- It is also unclear how several groups—such as pregnant women and those with certain diseases, as well as people who already had documented COVID-19 infections—will react to the vaccine since they were excluded from most studies.

* The goal of vaccination need not be the achievement of herd immunity, but rather to protect vulnerable people from COVID-19 and thus to reduce the incidence of serious disease and death.
* It is unclear if and when people may need to be revaccinated.
* It is unclear whether people who had COVID-19 and thus are naturally immune have any benefit, or any risk, from being vaccinated.
* There is no evidence that vaccinated individuals are at an increased risk of becoming sick from COVID-19 variants, based on observations in the community.
* There is no evidence that vaccinated individuals confer any benefit from masks, handwashing measures, or social distancing after they are immune.
* It appears the vaccinated individuals are very unlikely to spread COVID-19 to others.

Why a BRCT?

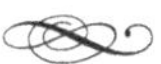

THE BRCT IS AN IMAGE that is worth a thousand words. It is based on an old English language adage meaning that "complex and sometimes multiple ideas can be conveyed by a single still image which conveys its meaning or essence more effectively than a mere verbal description." So, the general concept has been around for a while, but applying it to health issues like COVID-19 is a new concept.

In this book, which serves as a companion to our Springer Nature book on COVID-19 (to be published in August 2021) communication, we tried to validate the value of presenting medical data in a uniform, familiar, unambiguous, and easily graspable format. We demonstrated in an earlier book, *Interpreting Health Benefits and Risks*, how a BRCT theater format can help patients understand the risks and benefits of virtually all health decisions that they may have to make.

When information is given to them in a theater, when it is accurate and uniform, when both risks and benefits of interventions are provided, then patients can make personalized decisions based on their own medical needs and their own preferences.

All of us see the medical world through a unique lens. Health care decisions can be frightening and complex; we don't want to make the wrong decision, and we are often bombarded by information that we cannot understand and which is not necessarily factual. The morass of misinformation, presented to us in a misleading way, can lead us to make decisions that are not consistent with our own preferences.

Whether our choices involve taking a certain medicine for high cholesterol, using a blood thinner for atrial fibrillation or a memory medicine for dementia, having a heart stent placed, or undergoing a certain test, all these decisions, if framed in the context of a BRCT, can be made more rationally and in a patient-centric way.

COVID-19 AND THE BRCT

During this very frightening and often confusing pandemic, medical communication has been misleading, conflicting, and often erroneous. We have shown in this book the value of using a visual aid to better demonstrate the risks of COVID-19 and the benefits/risks of some of our interventions. Two recent articles about COVID-19 communication, both of which were published in May 2021 as we were completing this book, highlight the value of our approach.

An <u>article</u> by David Leonhardt in the *New York Times* in May 2021 puts some of what we discussed in focus. The CDC issued new guidelines and suggested that less than 10 percent of COVID-19 transmission occurred outdoors. According to the author, "the number is almost certainly misleading." He adds, "Saying that less than 10 percent of COVID-19 transmission occurs outdoors is akin to saying that sharks attack fewer than 20,000 swimmers a year. (The actual worldwide number is around 150.) It's both true and deceiving. This isn't just a gotcha math issue. It is an example of how the CDC is struggling to communicate effectively, and leaving many people confused about what's truly risky."

In fact, according to Leonhardt, the actual chance of outdoor transmission is less than 1/1,000, or, if the CDC wanted to communicate accurately and understandably, one seat in a 1,000-seat theater, as shown below. That's only the transmission rate. The chance of getting sick from that transmission, or having enough virus to spread it, is far lower. Had the CDC used a BRCT to express risks, people and policymakers may have had a better sense of whether to be nervous outdoors or even whether they should be wearing a mask outdoors when risk is so low and when mask use (as we have shown) has no proven benefit. They can put themselves in the theater and better understand their own risk.

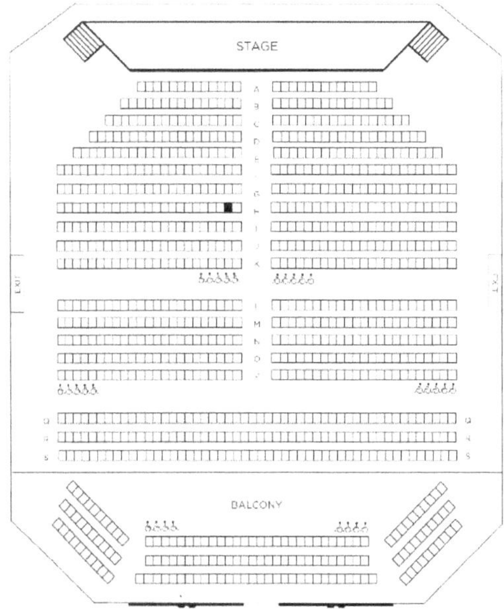

Also in May 2021, an <u>article</u> in *Science* by Adam Rogers called "The Statistical Secrets of COVID-19 Vaccines" similarly demonstrates how BRCTs can help people understand the risks and benefits of certain interventions. Rogers states that the messaging about vaccines isn't clear because the statistics tossed at the public by agencies and pharmaceutical companies are confusing and deceptive. Rather than using actual numbers and demonstrating how those numbers may benefit people based on their risk of dying of COVID-19, all that these agencies and companies did was to encourage mistrust in the vaccine process and promote vaccine hesitancy. "This pandemic has widely varying risks across populations, and those change over time," says Rogers. "By not being clear about the different flavors of risk and benefit for different vaccines and different people, public health experts have let doubt and dodgy personal interpretations flourish."

As we demonstrated with our **BRCTs** throughout this book, the risk of death of COVID-19 varies, and when that risk is compared to the benefits and risks of a vaccine, a person can make an informed decision about whether to get that vaccine.

We have confirmed, for example, that the risk of dying of COVID-19 differs dramatically between different demographic groups; for instance, the risk of a student dying of this virus is far less than the risks that students face every day, while the risk of an elder in long-term care dying is quite substantial, as shown in the BRCTs below. Such information can help individuals and policymakers make rational and personalized decisions based on data that is accurate and understandable, whether it is regarding vaccination or other interventions being used to slow viral spread.

Risk of a long-term care resident dying if they are infected with COVID-19 infection

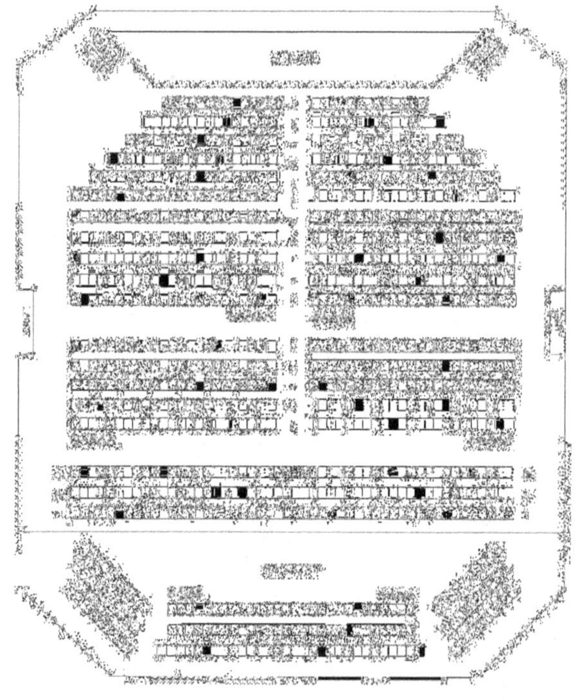

The average risk of someone not in long-term care dying if they are infected with COVID-19 infection; the difference in risk will vary based on age, as we show in chapter one

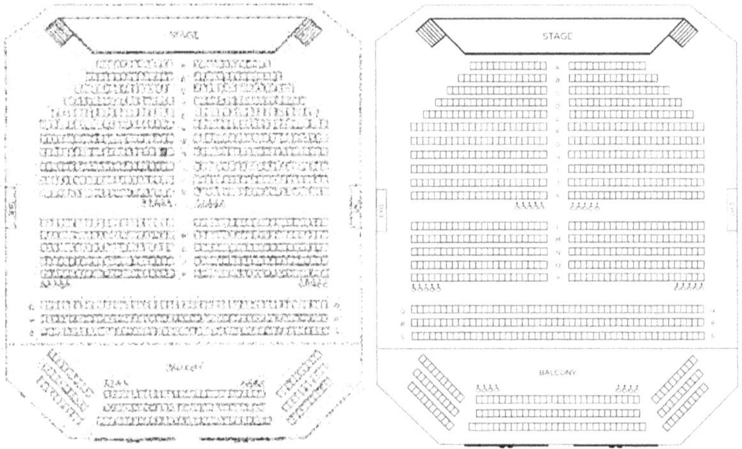

We have shown, too, what we know about the various "treatments" of the pandemic instated by public health officials and state governments, from school closings, to universal mask use, to global quarantines, to vaccination, to several medicine regimens. We have clarified that in some cases the risks and benefits of these interventions are known, but that in many more cases they are uncertain or vary based on different populations. Many statements made in a declarative way actually have no science to back them up, and this should be communicated to the public. Instead, many "experts" insist that certain interventions work, and then they change their minds just as quickly and just as confidently, all along presenting information in a misleading way. For instance, consider the following points:

* At the onset of the outbreak, the CDC and other agencies declared that masks don't help; then they shifted gears and stated that they do work; then they stated that we need two masks—never backing any of these declarations up by data which acknowledged

the uncertainty of masks use, which we have demonstrated in this book.

* Public health agencies put one-way aisles in stores and then took them away. They stated that you had to be six feet apart, then three feet; then they changed the distance based on where you are. None of this was backed up by facts and all of it is uncertain, something not ever stated by those "experts" and policymakers who insisted that everyone must comply.

* Schools and colleges were closed and remained closed for much of the spring and fall of 2020, and when they opened, restrictions remained that had no basis in scientific fact, but you wouldn't know that if you listened to "experts" and the media, all of whom denied the uncertainty of what they were declaring to be fact.

By using a BRCT to demonstrate what we don't know—which we have represented as a theater with a question mark—we can better understand what we do know. Not knowing how a certain intervention impacts those we are trying to help can guide us as to whether we should continue to use that intervention. Thus, the BRCT below is a powerful tool because it lets the public and policymakers understand where there is uncertainty, something that can guide decision-making.

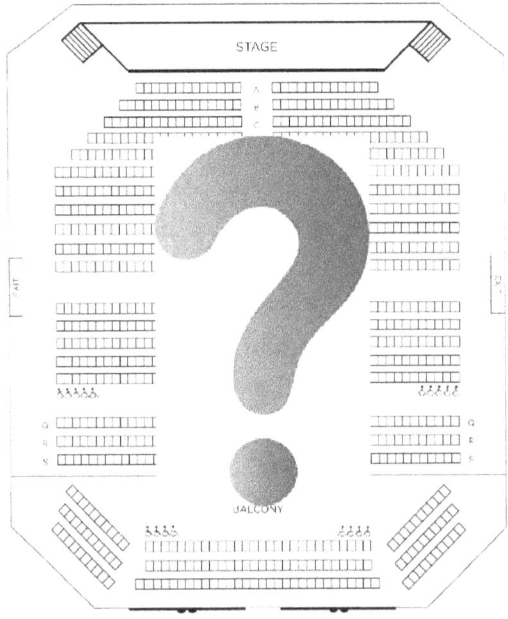

Far too often in the COVID-19 pandemic, those who have communicated to the public and established policy—from self-declared experts, to reporters, to public health officials, to government agencies, to political leaders—simply made declarative assertions that had no scientific basis. When policies were not working, or even if they may have caused harm, these experts did not relent or reconsider their approach, or even acknowledge the uncertainty of what they were doing; instead, they far too often continued to declare unequivocally that the treatments worked. Such erroneous and misleading communication led to untoward results and prevented both people and society from confronting COVID-19 in a sensible and effective way.

With a BRCT, we can factually demonstrate what we know, and also demonstrate what we don't know. We can show both the positive and negative ramifications of our interventions and also show which groups are most in need of our attention. None of that was done in the COVID-19 crisis, and in this book, we attempted to show how a BRCT-based approach can resolve that problem going forward.

How could we have reacted to our nursing home crisis had we relied on the BRCT model? We would have seen that the long-term care population was the most vulnerable to this virus, and we would have thus focused much more effort in this area. We would have acknowledged that we don't know if strict isolation and mask use resulted in any benefit or harm, and in the light of increasing COVID-19 and non-COVID-19 deaths and disability, we may have shifted gears. Maybe we would have demanded that a randomized trial be conducted to assess the efficacy of other strategies; maybe we would have simply tried something else, such as daily rapid testing or paying nursing home aides to stay overnight for several weeks so as to minimize their community carriage of disease.

Regardless of what we did next, the use of BRCTs could have allowed us to better understand the science behind our approaches, whether the BRCT showed benefits or risks, or whether it showed uncertainty of the outcome. Instead, many experts and policymakers simply trumpeted the certainty of their approach in the wake of uncertainty and continued to demand strict compliance to ineffective and potentially deleterious interventions, rather than changing directions and perhaps saving countless lives in the process. That is how a BRCT can help guide policy; with a BRCT we don't rely on myth, dogma, or speculation. We rely on what we know and what we don't know.

On an individual level, BRCTs can help people understand their personal risks and benefits and make informed decisions. Whether deciding about getting a vaccine, wearing a mask on a walk through the park, remaining isolated or willingly going outside or to a store or socializing with friends, or wondering whether it's safe to send your child to school, all of these can be best assessed when a person puts himself/herself in a theater that demonstrates the risk of COVID-19 to them, and the risks and benefits of varying interventions such as mask use and social isolation.

Whether in demonstrating the risks and benefits of health decisions we face every day or in helping us to grapple with COVID-19 on

an individual and policy level, the BRCT is an invaluable tool to help guide us to make decisions that are best for us.

All medical decisions are inherently uncertain; the last thing we need is to have that uncertainty augmented by confusing and often misleading statistics and "expert" declarations. All health outcomes can be put in a BRCT; if they can't, then it means that we don't fully understand them.

BRCTs can show us what we know and what we don't know; they can be individualized for each person and demographic, and they can help us assess both our own risk of a certain illness and also the risks and benefits of various interventions. We encourage their use moving forward, not only in COVID-19 and any other pandemics that hit our shores but also in the general realm of health care decision-making. **If COVID-19 showed us anything, it is that it's time we change course when it comes to medical communication.**

After seeing relevant information and data regarding COVID-19 risks, it's up to you to make the decision that you think is right for you.

LIST OF AGENCIES THAT PROVIDE INFORMATION TO THE PUBLIC REGARDING COVID-19:

- *Administration for Children and Families
- Administration for Community Living
- Advisory Council on Historic Preservation
- Appalachian Regional Commission
- Army Public Health Center
- Centers for Disease Control and Prevention
- Centers for Medicare and Medicaid
- Chief Human Capital Officers Council
- Consumer Financial Protection Bureau
- Consumer Product Safety Commission
- Corporation for National and Community Service
- Customs and Border Patrol
- Cybersecurity and Infrastructure Security Agency
- Defense Acquisition University
- Defense Commissary Agency
- Department of Agriculture
- Department of Defense
- Department of Defense Office of Financial Readiness
- Department of Education
- Department of Energy
- Department of Health and Human Services
- Department of Homeland Security
- Department of Housing and Urban Development
- Department of Labor
- Department of State
- Department of the Interior
- Department of the Treasury
- Department of the Treasury Inspector General
- Director of National Intelligence
- Drug Enforcement Administration Diversion Control Division

- Economic Development Administration
- Election Assistance Commission
- Environmental Protection Agency
- Equal Employment Opportunity Commission
- Export-Import Bank of the United States
- Farm Credit Administration
- Federal Aviation Administration
- Federal Bureau of Prisons
- Federal Communications Commission
- Federal Deposit Insurance Corporation
- Federal Emergency Management Agency (FEMA)
- Federal Reserve System
- Federal Student Aid
- Federal Trade Commission
- Federal Transit Administration
- Financial Crimes Enforcement Network
- Food and Drug Administration
- Forest Service
- General Services Administration
- Government Publishing Office
- Health Resources and Services Administration
- Indian Affairs
- Indian Health Service
- Institute of Museum and Library Services
- Inter-American Foundation
- Internal Revenue Service
- Legacy Management (Department of Energy)
- Maritime Administration
- Merit Systems Protection Board
- Military Community and Family Policy
- Military Health System
- National Aeronautics and Space Administration
- National Archives

- National Cancer Institute
- National Capital Planning Commission
- National Credit Union Administration
- National Finance Center
- National Institute of Environmental Health Sciences
- National Institute on Drug Abuse
- National Institutes of Health
- National Marine Sanctuaries
- National Park Service
- National Renewable Energy Laboratory
- National Science Foundation
- Navy and Marine Corps Public Health Center
- Nuclear Regulatory Commission
- Occupational Safety and Health Review Commission
- Office of Personnel Management
- Office of the Assistant Secretary for Preparedness and Response
- Office of the Comptroller of the Currency
- Pension Benefit Guarantee Corporation
- Railroad Retirement Board
- Small Business Administration
- Social Security Administration
- Substance Abuse and Mental Health Services Administration
- Tennessee Valley Authority
- Transportation Security Administration
- U.S. Agency for Global Media
- U.S. Agency for International Development
- U.S. Agency for International Development Office of Inspector General
- U.S. Census Bureau
- U.S. Citizenship and Immigration Service
- U.S. Copyright Office
- U.S. Fire Administration
- U.S. Merchant Marine Academy

- U.S. Northern Command
- U.S. Patent and Trademark Office
- U.S. Postal Inspection Service
- U.S. Postal Service (USPS)
- U.S. Special Operations Command
- U.S. Trade Representative
- Washington Headquarters Services
- White House

About the Authors

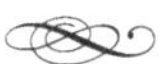

ANDY LAZRIS, MD, CMD IS board certified physician in Internal Medicine and a Certified Medical Director who runs a geriatric medical practice. He has written numerous fiction and nonfiction books, including *Curing Medicare* (Cornell University Press, 2014), and both *Interpreting Health Benefits and Risks* and *Utilizing Effective Risk Communication in COVID-19* with Erik Rifkin. He has a podcast and an ongoing blog, and gives frequent health-related talks in the community. He worked on the front lines during the COVID-19 pandemic in long term care.

Erik Rifkin, PhD is an environmental scientist who has had over 40 years of experience in characterizing human health and ecological risks from exposure to contaminants in soil, aquatic ecosystems, air and sediments. He has provided assistance and guidance to federal and state regulatory agencies, corporations, NGOs and the public in assessing risks. In addition to publishing articles in peer-reviewed science journals, Dr. Rifkin is a co-author of Springer Nature books: *The Illusion of Certainty-Health Benefits and Risks*, 2007; *Interpreting Health Benefits and Risks*, 2015; and, *Utilizing Effective Risk Communication in COVID-19* (publication scheduled for August, 2021). His professional activities have under-scored the importance of the communication of health risks and benefits to impacted groups.

Acknowledgments

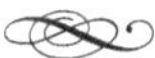

WE WOULD LIKE TO TAKE this opportunity to thank Kris Rifkin, a graphic designer, for her advice and guidance regarding the use of appropriate images to illustrate large numbers of people. Her assistance and responsiveness played an important role in developing appropriate graphics for communicating COVID-19 health risks and benefits.

We would also like to thank our editor at Amnet Systems.

References, Articles, and Videos

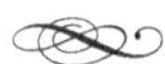

ALL REFERENCES USED IN THIS book, if not hyperlinked, can be found in our Springer Nature book Utilizing Effective Risk Communication in COVID-19.

The data we have used, unless indicated otherwise, is from the United States

We have links to our other books, our videos, and our articles at our website, www.doc-patient-talk.com

www.ingramcontent.com/pod-product-compliance
Lightning Source LLC
Chambersburg PA
CBHW050732260726
48661CB00001B/190